MISSING ME

MISSING ME

A MEMOIR OF POSTPARTUM PSYCHOSIS AND THE LONG ROAD BACK

AYANA LAGE

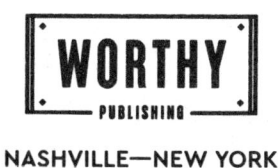

NASHVILLE—NEW YORK

Copyright © 2026 by Ayana Lage
Cover design by Kristen Paige Andrews
Cover copyright © 2026 by Hachette Book Group, Inc.

To protect their privacy, the names and identifying details of certain people included in this memoir have been changed.

Hachette Book Group supports the right to free expression and the value of copyright. The purpose of copyright is to encourage writers and artists to produce the creative works that enrich our culture.

The scanning, uploading, and distribution of this book without permission is a theft of the author's intellectual property. If you would like permission to use material from the book (other than for review purposes), please contact Permissions@hbgusa.com. Thank you for your support of the author's rights.

Worthy Books
Hachette Book Group
1290 Avenue of the Americas
New York, NY 10104
worthypublishing.com
X.com/WorthyPub

First Edition: March 2026

Worthy Books is a division of Hachette Book Group, Inc. The Worthy Books name and logo are trademarks of Hachette Book Group, Inc.

The publisher is not responsible for websites (or their content) that are not owned by the publisher.

The Hachette Speakers Bureau provides a wide range of authors for speaking events. To find out more, go to hachettespeakersbureau.com or email HachetteSpeakers@hbgusa.com.

Library of Congress Cataloging-in-Publication Data

Name: Lage, Ayana author
Title: Missing me : a memoir of postpartum psychosis and the long road back / Ayana Lage.
Description: First edition. | Nashville : Worthy Books, 2026. | Includes bibliographical references.
Identifiers: LCCN 2025038962 | ISBN 9781546008958 hardcover | ISBN 9781546008965 trade paperback | ISBN 9781546008972 ebook
Subjects: LCSH: Lage, Ayana | Puerperal psychoses—Patients—United States—Biography | African American mothers—Biography | Puerperal Psychoses—Religious aspects | Faith—Psychology | LCGFT: Autobiographies
Classification: LCC RG851 .L34 2026
LC record available at https://lccn.loc.gov/2025038962

ISBNs: 978-1-546-00895-8 (hardcover); 978-1-546-00897-2 (ebook); 978-1-668-65378-4 (audio)

Printed in Canada

MRQ-T

10 9 8 7 6 5 4 3 2 1

For Nora and Elliott

CONTENTS

Introduction: The Book Has Unhinged Parts   ix

CHAPTER ONE	My Broken Brain	1
CHAPTER TWO	Miracles	21
CHAPTER THREE	Raising Hell	35
CHAPTER FOUR	The Worst Day	49
CHAPTER FIVE	A Mother's Love	65
CHAPTER SIX	I Got Lucky	73
CHAPTER SEVEN	The Doctors Saved My Life	81
CHAPTER EIGHT	The Pretty Prophet	95
CHAPTER NINE	Not Scared	111
CHAPTER TEN	A Terrible Hangover	125
CHAPTER ELEVEN	Sitting in Silence	141
CHAPTER TWELVE	The Evidence	153
CHAPTER THIRTEEN	You Won't Be Here Forever	169

Acknowledgments   *181*
Notes   *185*
About the Author   *187*

INTRODUCTION

The Book Has Unhinged Parts

God told me I'd write this book. Well, kind of.

Nine days after giving birth to my daughter, I stood up and told my husband I had a prophecy to share. It was nighttime, and I'd been trying in vain to fall asleep when I suddenly heard a booming voice say something incredible. *I was going to be an author.* It was so loud that I almost covered my ears, but my husband looked unaffected. An adrenaline rush hit me like never before—it felt like electricity was running through my veins.

From the look on my husband's face after my announcement, I could tell he was concerned—we are not the kind of people who hear from God—but I was too excited to care. God was telling me secrets. Who wouldn't want to write a book? I felt deliriously happy.

I couldn't sleep that night because the prophecies wouldn't stop coming. Instead of getting much-needed rest, I blasted music from my phone and cried because I felt so inspired. I'd spent my whole life trying to figure God out, and he was finally giving me answers. I was so excited about my newfound spiritual gift that I told people he was speaking to me. I had an extensive support system—my husband, parents, sisters, doula, and a couple of close friends—all of whom I deeply trusted and all of whom started to think I needed medical help. My behavior was not explainable by postpartum blues.

The day after I started hearing God's voice, my husband and father drove me to a local hospital for an evaluation. I spent the entire drive muttering to myself. God's revelations were starting to freak me out. I was positive my family members were going to try to hurt my baby. I knew my daughter was going to die. I hated him for telling me these things, but I didn't want the words to stop. COVID-19 pandemic restrictions meant I had to go inside the hospital alone. I paced a cramped exam room, feeling increasingly disoriented as I yelled for help. The hallucinations started a few minutes later.

They diagnosed me with postpartum psychosis, and I didn't leave the hospital for seventeen days. During my stay, I filled up a stack of notebooks on a mission to rewrite the Bible. I hid them under my pillow, afraid that another patient would try to steal my prophecies while I slept. None of the medications I was prescribed were working, and it didn't help that I sometimes refused to swallow them. Hospital staff members would explain that the pills would make me feel better, but I didn't trust them. I would wake up, agitated as ever, and turn to my notebooks. The hospital told my husband I might need treatment at a long-term psychiatric care facility if I didn't improve.

Getting well enough to leave the hospital was a fight—don't worry, we'll get into that soon. But just know that it wasn't the most challenging part. When I got home, I had enough material to keep me in therapy for a lifetime. I wasn't physically or mentally present for my daughter's first month. I fell into a deep depression, wondering whether my early absence would cause problems down the road. I knew she had no memory of me being gone, but I wondered whether she somehow sensed it. What kind of mother can't take care of her baby?

When I was discharged from the psychiatric ward, they asked whether I wanted the nonsense-filled notebooks. I brought them home and shoved them under my bed. I was on a cocktail of antipsychotics and mood stabilizers that left me behaving erratically. I threw away half of my composition notebook collection one night for reasons I still don't understand. Why I didn't toss the whole stack is a mystery to me.

The remaining notebooks have been tucked away ever since. I keep them in a taped-up cardboard box neatly labeled HOSPITAL that acts as a bit of a 2020 time capsule. When you open it, you see used surgical masks, a reminder that I was hospitalized during the peak of the pandemic. I scrawled delusions on scraps of paper when I wasn't near a notebook, and they clutter the bottom of the box. There's even a half-empty bottle of hospital shampoo in there. It looks like it all belongs in the trash.

For a while, I viewed this hospital box the same way someone might approach a haunted house. I was fearful because I wasn't sure what was waiting in there, or how I'd react. I tried to push the notebooks out of my mind at first. But as much as I ran away from it, I couldn't avoid the totality of my experience. I needed to understand what happened to me to find a way forward. I was tempted to push it all out of mind, but a part of me wanted—needed—to know the gory details.

But before we get into all that, here's one thing I want to say.

You can be prepared for something hard, even excruciating. You can scan Reddit and Wirecutter and TikTok for all the advice and recommendations in the world. You can be the friend who always has a plan if things go wrong. But what happens when you completely lose touch with reality? What do you do? As a survivor of psychosis, making sense of my lived experience was so much harder than I anticipated. And a question plagued me.

Could I find answers in the box?

Postpartum psychosis is often associated with infanticide. It's not hard to angrily wonder what kind of parent could hurt their child—but once you hear the voices yourself, there's a perspective shift. These women are not villains. Often, they believe they're protecting their children, like any good parent would. I easily could've been one of them.

The social stigma of psychosis wasn't even the worst part for me—it was my own struggle to understand. I knew nearly nothing about the condition before I lived it, and I found myself desperately reading books and scouring Google as I tried to recover. It was something that had happened to me without my permission, and I felt violated by it all. And then there was the issue of my embarrassing behavior leading up to my mental break. People liking me is all I've ever wanted, but psychosis didn't care.

I had religious delusions to unpack, too. I'm a Pentecostal preacher's kid, so I know something about listening for God's voice. But in the years leading up to my psychotic episode, I'd walked away from fundamentalist faith. I wasn't quite sure what I thought of religion. The version of myself that emerged while I was sick is hard to comprehend: a fire-and-brimstone preacher offering prophecies to anyone on the psych ward floor who wanted one. I was never more powerful in my life. Nothing else mattered.

When I left the hospital, I marveled at how quiet it was inside my head. Part of me missed the chaos—being able to ask God anything I wanted: Will I write a book one day? Is the hospital staff trying to kill me? Who's going to win the 2020 election?—and get an answer right away. *(The responses I heard, in order: Yes, yes, Joe Biden. In fairness, I had a fifty-fifty chance with that last one.)* I understand why people consciously choose not to take needed psychiatric medication. When I was in psychosis, I was unstoppable.

Many elements are missing when I try to piece together the days before and during my psychotic episode. I've always prided myself on being a reliable narrator, but this was one scenario when I couldn't always trust my memory. I requested my hospital records soon after my release, an idea my loved ones vehemently opposed. But without them, all I had to understand my experience was fractured memories, other people's recollections, and my cryptic scribbles. The records did give me answers, some of which I wasn't ready to hear. My relationship with them is complicated—we'll get to that, too.

Thinking about my psychosis used to be uncomfortable for me, and it felt safest to leave that chapter of my life behind rather than dwell on it, let alone write about it. I wasn't sure I wanted postpartum psychosis to be the first thing that came up when someone googled me. But the more I considered it all, the more I realized that my openness could shed light on the condition. I started to tell friends and family about my experience. People didn't always know what to say, but I felt less ashamed once I got honest, awkwardness be damned. I began to think about how much of my story I wanted to share with the world. So I started to write and—this is the crucial part—returned to the box of notebooks.

The scribbles are barely coherent. But when I flip through them, I recall the delusions that sparked the words. There are pages devoted to my false beliefs that someone was trying to hurt my daughter and that the hospital was running experiments on patients. I remember a lot of it vividly but don't recall some parts, although I can picture myself in the psych ward's common room, alternating between marker and pencil as I wrote as quickly as possible. When I first looked at the notebooks, I didn't know whether I'd shake it off as nonsense. But when I combined them with what I remembered from the time, I started to get a clearer picture—one that I'm sharing with you. The italicized portions of this book are pulled from the journals, hospital records, and my memory.

I was surprised at how relevant many of the words felt to me. Of course, there was a lot that I had to ignore, like the pages dedicated to debating whether I was dead or alive or stuck in hell without an escape route. Still, there are bits that I realized applied to my life outside the hospital. Some moments were a comforting reminder that I didn't lose myself entirely. This introduction's title—and that of several other chapters in this book—are inspired by my psych ward journals. *Missing Me* is a look into the events leading up to my break from reality and what came after. The pages that follow are honest, heartfelt, and, at times, a bit unhinged.

Let's dive in.

MISSING ME

CHAPTER ONE

My Broken Brain

The patient is a 27-year-old black female admitted to the Behavioral Health Unit. The patient was grossly psychotic, delusional, confused, paranoid.
 —My Clinical Documentation Record, page 87

Author's note: This chapter contains mentions of self-harm and suicidal ideation.

I stare at the ceiling in my bedroom, my eyes filled with silent tears. I am so happy. God has chosen me to write a book—a bestseller, no less. My days will soon be filled with television interviews and a splashy tour. Everyone will read the book once it's published. He reveals that it's a success because it's free of charge. Wait. How will I pay for the tour if the book is free? He chides me for worrying. "I will provide," he says. I'm already accustomed to his voice, and it's only been a few minutes since the first prophecy. Or maybe it's been hours.

Let's rewind.

I am in bed, trying to fall asleep. My husband says he is very concerned. Apparently, I haven't slept in days. I don't want to lie next to him, but there aren't any other beds in the house. He can't be trusted, especially since he told me I shouldn't be alone with my nine-day-old baby. It's barbaric. I prefer to stay awake to keep an eye on him, watching as he makes a bottle for my daughter. Besides, I like how quiet everything is at nighttime. Last night, I watched Supermarket Sweep reruns for hours, wondering whether the show was real. I still don't know.

My mind wanders. I feel myself drifting off and try to fight it. Then, I hear a chime so loud it hurts my ears. I see a too-bright light bulb. I squint.

There's a roaring voice—almost thunderous. "YOU WILL WRITE A BOOK, AND IT WILL BE THE MOST SUCCESSFUL ONE TO EVER BE PUBLISHED," it booms.

I forgive my husband; the news is too good to keep to myself. I rush the words out, and he looks at me anxiously. I am annoyed that he doesn't get it. Thankfully, my parents are here to help with the baby. Someone needs to understand the gravity of my newfound calling. I yell for them and shout the heavenly word I've received. They, too, look troubled.

Soon, my husband is falling asleep next to me. It hurts my feelings. How can he not stay awake during the most significant moment of my life? If I can't talk to him, I'll talk to God. Why would God wait until the baby's birth to start speaking? "We have a lot going on right now," I whisper. "You could've revealed this to me a few months ago."

The dismay quickly passes. I ask him to tell me secrets about my favorite people. He starts to share it all. I scroll through Spotify, tap the first Christian worship playlist I see, and grab a notepad to keep track of all he's saying.

This is how it starts.

The first episode arrives before puberty.

I am lightheaded. My limbs tingle. My heart races, and I am disoriented. My bedroom walls are closing in on me. I cannot catch my breath. I am trapped in someone else's body, and there's no way to escape. My loved ones are suddenly strangers. Then, the terror subsides, and I am overwhelmed by confusion. I check the time. Only a few minutes have passed. I would've bet my iPod that it had been hours. I have heard talk about crazy people before. Maybe this is how it begins. The anxiety rises to my throat when I think about it, so I brush it off and block it all from memory. I have no choice but to move on and hope it was a fluke. I make it a few days before it happens again. *Oh no, oh no, oh no.*

This, I will eventually learn, is called a panic attack. I will learn to live with the terror, even though I am only eleven years old.

FIFTEEN YEARS BEFORE

I turn the bathtub handle to the left and wait for the water to warm. It's been a year since the attacks started, and they are worse when I am alone. I consider skipping showers to avoid the terrifying moment I realize another episode is on its way but worry I'll stink. Instead, I improvise, taking a *Sweet Valley High* book into the bathroom to prevent even a second of solitude. I shrug when my mother finds a soggy paperback in my room and offer no explanation. The anxiety begins to take even more from me. My grades slip. My family becomes used to my moodiness—the anxiety makes me emotional. It is all chalked up to prepubescent angst. I am the only one who knows I'm falling apart, and the weight is too much to bear.

I do not know how far things will go. I am twelve when I sit by Crystal on the school bus, the empty seat beckoning. She has strawberry-blonde hair and a Southern twang when she speaks. She tells me she just moved to the neighborhood from Kentucky. I like her immediately. When my parents meet her, they are wary for reasons they do not articulate. I do not care. Her home life isn't great, and I try to comfort her as best a twelve-year-old can. One day, out of the blue, she whispers that she knows how to disassemble a razor to get to the blade inside. I do it sometimes, she tells me. It helps with everything. This intrigues me. I've just hit puberty and have started shaving my legs. I have a razor. I can figure it out. Harming myself is a new thought, but the anxiety leaves me desperate to feel something. There's no downside, I think.

I cannot ignore the release I feel when I see blood. I will forget the gory details—for once, my brain keeps me safe—but the relief is immediate. I am ashamed, of course. Who wouldn't be? I know better. My behavior humiliates me. I am unable to fully commit—too scared to cut deeply—but the shallow wounds I create still provide comfort. Dabbing my arms with toilet paper becomes normal; wearing long sleeves on the hottest Florida days until the cuts disappear is a frequent practice. We all self-sabotage in different ways. Mine happened to be violent.

A few months after I meet my friend, I draft a suicide note. Instead of paying attention to my science teacher droning on about the periodic table, I brainstorm the best way to kill myself. My eight-year-old sisters can't be the ones who find me. I raise my hand and ask to go to the bathroom. I lock myself into a stall and sob. I am too young to watch PG-13 movies but old enough to crave the end.

My parents keep me safe. They will do anything for me. My father once looked at me with serious eyes and said, "You won't ever get in trouble for telling us something we wouldn't have found out ourselves." Years later, I will joke that they are the one topic that doesn't come up in therapy. Their door is always open. Like the time when I was ten years old and looking for a hobby.

I attempt tennis before deciding I don't like to sweat. Then comes piano lessons; I do not have the discipline to practice at home. I take a stab at cheerleading before realizing I'm not flexible enough to do a forward roll. Eventually, I decide that my passion is spending time online. No one acknowledges the absurdity. On the Christmas tree that year, three ornaments signal our interests: a basketball for one sister, a gymnast for the other, and a tiny computer to represent my love of the internet.

We go on yearly vacations. Birthday parties are gorgeous affairs. Nightly family dinners around the kitchen table are a requirement. My parents would leap into action if they knew. But they aren't mind readers, and I do an impressive job convincing them and everyone else that nothing is seriously wrong with me. I cannot tell them this. Even if I wanted to, how on earth would I find the words?

One of my friends—a child herself—senses that I am in danger. She tells the school counselor, who calls my parents. Their faces are etched with concern when they find out. It's every parent's worst fear. You will do anything to keep your child safe. But how do you protect them from themselves? I start therapy for the first time, and it will not be the last.

I am cagey with the therapist—no one can know about the panic attacks. My report card comes back with a failing grade for the first time. I have disappointed everyone. The school year ends. I strive to be better and find my footing as a bright, outgoing child. I beg my parents to take me to the mall; my clothes are now from Hollister and Abercrombie & Fitch. Dorky eyeglasses are tossed in favor of contacts. I weasel into the eighth-grade popular crowd and feel like I've figured it all out. The Fabulous Five, four of my closest friends and I call ourselves. I will never feel lonely again.

The panic attacks still happen. I am suffocating.

I do not know what to do.

About 2 percent of adolescents experience panic disorder in their lifetime.[1] I have never been particularly fortunate.

When I am nine, my parents take away my library card as a punishment for misbehaving. It is more effective than depriving me of television. Reading is the only escape I have. I wander the stacks, savoring the smell of the books in the young adult section. The library allows me to check out thirty-five books at a time. This delights me. I fall down Wikipedia rabbit holes and file away obscure, useless facts that never come up in conversation. No one is surprised when I decide I will one day be a journalist.

I love to learn, but that does not apply to what's happening in my brain. I cope by avoiding the topic. When I tell my therapist that our sessions have made me feel much better, she looks pleased with herself. My convincing answers allow me to coast through until she says I no longer need to come. It is easy to figure out what people want to hear, even as a child. I am happy to be done.

It takes me years to find the courage to google what I am experiencing. Once I decide to do research, I cannot quite find the words. My hands shake as I type in phrases like "suddenly feeling confused" and "trapped in someone else's body." None of the results ever resonate. I learn about dissociative episodes when I am eighteen. It is the first time I feel close to having an answer.

I scroll through an article about dissociative identity disorder, hoping this is it. There are some commonalities between my panic attacks and the symptoms spelled out on my screen, but it doesn't feel right. I don't meet the diagnostic criteria for the condition, once known as multiple personality disorder. Someone with dissociative identity disorder has separate, distinct identities that they transition between. This isn't a struggle of mine. I give up. Maybe I am the first person in the world to go through this. I've spent too much time thinking about it, I tell myself. My curiosity might trigger an episode.

I watch old episodes of *House* when I am bored. I dream of a deadpan but brilliant physician who can figure out why I am going crazy, all in a forty-five-minute television episode. My desire for a doctor to fix things isn't desperate enough to make me see one. I frantically try to pinpoint what is wrong on my own. I am better equipped to deal with the complexities of mental health as a newly minted adult than I was at eleven years old, but I still lack the language to articulate what is happening to me. I finally work up the courage to tell someone.

I am driving home from college one night with my phone in my lap and my boyfriend on speakerphone. I take a big breath before rushing out the secret I've been holding in—that I have struggled with panic for years. That it's getting worse, and I don't see a way out. A long pause. "I love you," he says. "But I don't feel equipped to help you." I regret opening up in the first place. He gently asks if I've considered therapy. I take it as an insult.

The call ends, and I am furious with myself for my vulnerability. But a seed has been planted. I trust him more than anyone. He's one of the smartest people I know. If he thinks that I need to seek help, I might need it. Some part of me is desperate enough to believe him.

A few weekends later, I am at my parents' house, the same place where the terror first began. I ask them for help finding someone to talk to, rushing through the question so fast that my words are hard to separate. They are my first call when I have a scary decision. I can't imagine finding a therapist on my own. I'm only nineteen, after all.

They send me the counselor's name, and I make the appointment. I adore her from the first time we meet. She's a licensed mental health intern in her late twenties—old enough to be authoritative but young enough to feel relatable. It is essential that she likes me, too. She is a Christian, and we open and close our sessions with prayer. I finally feel at ease. She explains things in a way that makes sense. I open up.

My boyfriend and parents know that I am in therapy, but they still don't know how bad things really are. When I randomly burst into tears, I tell them school is causing me to freak out. My parents suggest taking fewer credit hours the following semester; I nod, unsure how to explain that one fewer class on my schedule will not solve any of my problems. My trusted therapist knows I struggle, but she is the only one, and even she doesn't know the full intensity and severity. I can't cause unnecessary concern by being dramatic. Plenty of people have it worse than I do. It does not occur to me that I might need someone—anyone—to worry about me.

I try to hide from the flashing cameras and paparazzi who yell my name, but they exhaust me. My hand shakes as I raise it to shield my eyes, and I cower in a spot in the corner of the room. I must shrink myself till I disappear. Every news organization in the world wants a piece of me—from the huge ones I've admired for years to tiny blog sites that receive no web traffic. I have always wondered what fame might feel like. I used to watch American Idol *in envy of ordinary people who become superstars overnight. Now that it is happening to me, I hate it.*

Everyone has questions for me. Actually, they have questions for God. I am the only person on the planet with direct access to him, and the crowds will not leave me alone until I pass along their inquiries. I wake up. Or maybe I was never sleeping? I am not sure. Is this all real, or is it a heavenly vision I need to interpret?

Only God knows, and he's not ready to tell me. I flip my thin pillow over and try to go back to sleep.

SEVEN YEARS BEFORE

When I hang up the phone, I feel like I'm dreaming. The man on the other end of the line has offered a journalism internship at one of the state's best newspapers. I'm a twenty-year-old student, and it is a dream come true. I text my family excitedly. Things are looking up.

Later that week, I am hospitalized for suicidal ideation.

The fake-it-till-you-make-it strategy I developed as a teenager gets me far. I take advanced courses throughout high school and leave with honors, giving a rousing graduation speech to my classmates. I move into my college apartment full of hope. Soon, I join student organizations and rush a sorority, all while obsessing over my grade point average. I am in love with the long-distance boyfriend who got me into therapy, and I feel confident we'll get married one day. I am not just normal. I am thriving.

My mental health episodes have not gone away, but I am so busy that they faze me less. Between classes, sorority events, extracurricular activities, and planning visits with my boyfriend, I barely have time to shower and sleep. I've finally cracked the code.

I take my last semester final on a Monday in early December, excited for the upcoming holiday. On the one-and-a-half-hour drive home, things start to crumble. I feel like the little girl of my youth, waiting for the anxiety to choke me again. My boyfriend suggests a casual date to cheer me up when I tell him I don't feel well. I run out of the coffee shop weeping for reasons I can't describe. The next day, I can barely get out of bed. The panic attacks are relentless, and the coping mechanisms are not working. I try to journal. I attempt to pray. My stomach relaxes as I exhale after deep breaths. Nothing gives me more than a few minutes of relief.

I force myself to daydream about the future and wonder whether I am dealing with seasonal blues that will go away when the sun doesn't set so early. Accepting the journalism internship—and watching the social media likes roll in after I share the news on Facebook—is a welcome distraction. But I cannot escape an uncomfortable truth: I am not sure I'll make it to the summer.

I have hidden how bad things are from my family, friends, and therapist for almost a decade. My mind is tired of pretending. Staying in my pajamas and refusing to eat is a relief. Allowing myself to collapse feels like surrender. I no longer have it in me to go through the motions. Everyone is terribly concerned. The attention feels comforting.

My mother brings me a slice of toast and gingerly asks how I am. The dam breaks, and I say the word *suicidal* aloud for the first time in years. Things move quickly. It is time to go to the emergency room.

I fidget in the car on the thirty-minute drive and balk at the imposing hospital building. I do not know what to expect. When I picture a psychiatric ward, I think of the stuff you see in horror movies. Will I be safe? Once inside, I change into a too-small gown and wait, willing myself to stay calm.

The hospital exam room is cold, and I shiver. Finally, someone is in here with me. The nurse speaks in a gentle tone and runs through a questionnaire to evaluate my mental well-being. I rate my depression and anxiety levels. She asks if I'm having thoughts of hurting myself; my face gives the answer. Then, she asks me something absurd. "Do you ever hear things that other people cannot hear?" I say no. She follows up with, "Have you ever received secret messages from the radio or television?" I almost laugh but manage to restrain myself. It makes me nervous, though—I'm not sure I want to be around the kind of patients who talk back to the TV.

When my concerned boyfriend enters the room, it is one of the first things I tell him. They asked if I've heard secret messages! Things could always be worse for me.

I do not stop to consider the people who say yes to the questions. There isn't room for them in my mind because I'm afraid. What might it be like to have a television anchor speak directly to me? Would it feel intoxicating to turn on the radio and hear personalized messages? Thankfully, it does not matter. I will never need to know.

Conditions like schizophrenia and psychosis are far more serious than what I'm dealing with—and way more intense. I think about when I walked out of a trendy sushi restaurant downtown and noticed an unhoused person walking, muttering to herself. She probably has a mental health condition, I thought with pity, but not in the same way that I do.

Here's what I believe: I'll never experience anything more serious than a panic attack. Although I should be more receptive to understanding the conditions I deem shameful, my approach doesn't affect my personal life. After all, the idea of someone like me—the same woman a therapist once half-jokingly called a control freak—going off the deep end is laughable. I am many things, but I'm not that far gone. The thought brings me more comfort than it should.

The hospital is clean and quiet, unlike the prison I've pictured. Patients usually have to share rooms, but I am fortunate to get my own. The friendly nurses let my family stay past visiting hours, so I never feel too alone. I am not supposed to have my phone, but my boyfriend lets me use his. I snap a picture of him in the visiting room, wanting to remember the terrible moment. He wears a blue shirt and eyeglasses. His smile is soft, and his eyes are full of worry. I commit it to memory.

For the first time since the panic attacks and self-harm started haunting me, I will be treated by doctors. The on-duty physician is clever and attentive. Her name is Dr. Lewis. She raises an eyebrow when I tell her the Christian therapist hasn't ever suggested seeing a psychiatrist for treatment. I have never considered this as a possibility. I am protective of my counselor. Maybe she didn't know, either. The doctor tells me medication will help me. She prescribes two of them. I am terrified of the potential side effects after we review them together. One of the drugs can cause suicidal thoughts, which seems odd—isn't that the reason I'm here in the first place? But the effect that scares me the most is weight gain. My relationship with my body is awful, and I worry this will worsen things. I fear fatness more than losing my life.

Through my fear, I decide to lean on Dr. Lewis. Three days later, I leave the hospital with the medications and shiny diagnoses. Within weeks, the fog starts to lift. I take a doctor's note explaining my condition to the disability resource center at school. My friends help me ease back into my busy schedule. This is the best I've ever felt.

I wrestle with who to tell about it all—the hospitalization, the new drugs, the psychologist and psychiatrist I am seeing. I try to remember that opening myself up to scrutiny may backfire. But I cannot ignore the pull to share my story with more people, which is ironic for someone so dedicated to hiding. For an inexplicable reason, the pendulum swings hard in the opposite direction.

I am so grateful I wish I could shout from a mountaintop, "Medication saved me!" I have never had qualms about baring my life to the world, and I jokingly call myself a chronic oversharer. In seventh grade, I listed all the boys I had crushes on and published it in my public Xanga web journal. (Hello to Josh H., if you're reading this.) Very little is sacred to me. I am a great secret keeper, but I do not have many. Still, I don't know whether people will be receptive. Am I an attention seeker? Do I want pity? I don't have an answer.

SIX YEARS BEFORE

I sit on the blue and orange patchwork quilt that covers the bed in my college apartment and take a big gulp of water. I reach for the bottle of small yellow pills on my nightstand and dump one into my hand. As I swallow, I think about how much better I feel. I can't believe it took me this long to get help. If I'd talked about this earlier, I might have improved without needing to be away from my family and friends. But the doctors were kind and dedicated to finding a solution for me. I feel happy that I finally have the care I need.

My mind wanders. How much better would my life be if I'd started taking psychiatric medication when I was fifteen and hiding in my room so no one knew I was panicking? Or at twelve, when my self-harm practice reached its peak? Even at nineteen, when I started seeing the therapist?

There's an uncomfortable truth. My lifelong refusal to acknowledge mental health may have stopped me from taking medication anyway. If nothing is wrong with you and you don't need help, why would you go to a psychiatrist? I am not antidrug, but I've always been a little afraid of them. At the hospital, I take the medicine they hand me in a small plastic cup. The nurse waits to make sure I swallow before I hand the cup back. I have struggled to get pills down my entire life and have to hide them in applesauce even as an adult. But on the ward, I quickly adapt and choke them down with water. I have no choice.

After my release, I dig into my old therapist's background and find that she incorporates biblical principles into her treatment plans. I squirm uncomfortably. Would a secular therapist have benefited me from the start? My Bible is dog-eared and filled with notes, so of course I'd love a Christian therapist. (This will change, but I do not know it yet.) I wonder whether she believes in medication at all. Why did she give me homework assignments when I needed Zoloft? When Dr. Lewis recommended finding a licensed psychologist instead of a mental health intern, I felt sad. Part of me wonders how she's doing. If she misses me. I shake off the thoughts.

As I climb under the sheets that night, I cannot stop thinking about the medications. I suspect I will need psychiatric drugs for the rest of my life—or at least for a very long time. I try to reframe my thinking. Science is so cool, I tell myself. Tiny pills barely bigger than my fingernail are resetting my brain chemistry. Truthfully, I am not quite sure how it works. Taking five seconds a day to swallow a tablet is a small price to pay. I want to believe this.

In my youth, I ran from my thoughts. I only confronted my mental health when my body left me no other option. What would have happened if I hadn't gone to the hospital that day over Christmas break? The morning of my admission, I had developed a plan to kill myself. My parents decided to hospitalize me. I am not sure I would have made it out alive otherwise, but I cannot fall into a "what if" rabbit hole. I go to sleep.

It takes me a year to put aside my fears and publicly write about what I experienced. I post a Facebook status right before the first anniversary of the hospitalization.

"One year ago today, I accepted a dream internship," it starts. I launch into the details of my hospitalization.

I explain my fear that people will assume I'm after their sympathy. I say that I'm willing to risk it if I'm able to start a frank conversation about mental health. "Depression doesn't rob me of feeling good about myself," I write. "It stops me from feeling anything at all."

The post ends with me saying I'm glad to share if my story helps even one person. After I click the post button, I close my web browser and try not to think about what I've done. I thoroughly documented my summer internship in social media posts. To onlookers, it seemed like I was living a dream. Letting people in on the truth is terrifying. When I find the courage to open Facebook again, the likes and comments are pouring in—and though I don't post hoping for any measure of virality, the positive feedback is comforting. Later, I will be proud of the version of myself who managed to swallow fear and share her experience.

I don't know it, but this is one of the most pivotal moments of my life. I have spent years desperately trying to ignore my mental health problems, and they've caught up to me. Compartmentalizing became second nature in my childhood, but I am changing things as an adult. Mental health is no longer a skeleton in the closet that brings embarrassment. I am not hiding but instead choosing to share the depths of my soul with anyone willing to listen. I feel overjoyed to finally have an answer and want others to feel that way, too. I am glad that I am not losing my mind, that my condition is treatable.

During this crucial time of self-discovery, I publish things I wouldn't put out into the world today. But that's expected when sharing your life online in your early twenties. I don't begrudge my younger self for not always getting it right.

Soon, I'm all in. I educate myself on mental health and barriers to treatment. My own path is straightforward enough—after the hospital, I begin outpatient treatment with the psychiatrist who saw me while I was admitted. I don't realize my luck. Having a mental health condition in the United States is an expense many cannot afford. I struggle enough even with the resources at my disposal; what would my care look like if I lacked family support? I can't believe so many people have to go into debt to take care of their mental health—or not receive treatment at all. My parents paid over $2,000 out of pocket for my hospital stay. The psychologist I adore doesn't accept health insurance. Between that and my prescriptions, my mother and father shell out $400 every month for my mental healthcare—an expense that I can't swing as a college student. I'm not sure what I would do without them. Mental healthcare saves me, but so do they.

Proudly calling myself a mental health advocate, I donate to relevant causes and write articles to help end the stigma. From the outside, it seems like I've found a higher purpose.

Don't get me wrong—I have. But there's something I won't ever say aloud because I feel guilty even thinking about it: I am glad that my mental health conditions are palatable ones. I remember reading about dissociative identity disorder back when I was trying to self-diagnose and imagining how terrifying it'd be to have something *really* wrong with me. My panic attacks and the times I struggle to get out of bed can be debilitating, but I don't feel embarrassed. Most important to me, I never lose touch with reality. Even during my worst moments, I keep my wits.

As I talk about mental health, I meet people with a variety of struggles—plenty who struggle with depression and anxiety like I do, along with obsessive-compulsive disorder, bipolar disorder, and other conditions. I educate myself as much as I can, but I secretly feel grateful for my diagnosis. People only see the parts of me that I deem acceptable to share. And I find success partly because of my anxiety-driven perfectionism.

My brain chemicals may be imbalanced, but I'm not crazy. This isn't how an advocate—someone who truly gets it—views mental health. I know that deep down, and I have the decency to feel ashamed.

I am no longer mentally ill because I am Jesus's favorite.

God is mad, but Jesus still cares about me. For the first time in my life, I can think clearly. It's like the time I saw an eye doctor when I was eight years old, and he prescribed eyeglasses. The fuzzy shapes I am accustomed to are suddenly sharp when I put the glasses on. I look out the car window in wonder on the drive home, marveling at the branches on the trees.

This is that, but infinitely better.
The bad news: I am in a coma.
The good news is that I am more lucid than ever.

The hospital nurses look at me dismissively when I tell them. But wait. How can I talk to people while comatose? Shouldn't I be unconscious? Signs and wonders abound, I think. God is so good to me, even though I'm mad at him right now. I will spend the rest of eternity praising him—if I can make it out of hell, that is.

CHAPTER TWO

Miracles

She has a fixed delusion that Satan has possessed her body and wants to kill her.
　　　—My Clinical Documentation Record, page 209

I scrawl "I need to see my baby" on a scrap of paper with a stubby pencil. My handwriting is slanted and hurried. The words will escape me if I don't get them out fast enough.

The baby in question is my daughter. Or maybe she isn't? I ask God whether I've imagined her. He reassures me that she's the second coming of Jesus. I smile.

My mind is gone. My grasp on reality is severed. But the baby—at least, the idea of her—is enough to keep me going. I feel a primal pull.

This is not the first time my brain has betrayed me.

SIXTEEN YEARS BEFORE

Streetlights are all that illuminate the room. The house is quiet; my family traded good nights and I love you's hours ago. I couldn't focus on my sixth-grade math worksheets earlier—all I've been thinking about is this moment. Finally, this is my chance. I whisper, even though no one can hear me. "God," I mumble, "I need you to deliver me." I sprinkle in words about how good he is for good measure, like I hear people do at church. Is God a bit vain for expecting this of me? I shake the thought and force myself to repent on the spot, hoping he won't send me to hell for my blasphemy.

No one knows about my anxiety but him. Sometimes, we talk for hours. Well, I do. I've been praying since before I learned my ABCs. I thank him for his provisions and ask him to nourish my body before every meal. It seems like communicating with God and hearing his response is second nature for everyone but me. My eyes open slowly when I think I've sufficiently begged him. My bubble-gum-pink bedroom looks the same. Has anything changed? I ask for a divine sign that he has healed me. I'm met with silence. I fall asleep, wondering whether I will experience the supernatural phenomenon I'm chasing. The following day, I have a panic attack. Rinse and repeat.

My prayers start to feel useless. The all-knowing God who supposedly loves me more than anything isn't listening. I am frantic. My Sunday school teachers tell me he built the whole world in six days. Why won't he help me? After my heart rate settles and I don't think I'm going to die anymore, I remind myself that I'm going to do great things. Why else would the devil try so hard to stop me? God and Satan are constantly at war, and my mind is a casualty. Not everyone has proof they'll one day change the world, but I'm one of the fortunate ones. This is part of my testimony. The Bible contains countless accounts of figures who faced hardship and came out on top.

My life will tell the same story.

When someone at church is sick, we surround them with arms outstretched, wailing as we declare they'll be made whole. During Sunday services, people are quick to jump to their feet and tearfully praise God for a disease that's disappeared. So-called signs and wonders are so ordinary that they're no longer surprising. When people stand up in church and thank God for healing their minds, I sit up straighter and listen closer. I have tangible proof that he's willing to fix people's anxiety. I don't need a therapist or even my parents. God's going to get me out of this.

I devour Scripture in search of answers. Part of me wonders whether I'm struggling to receive the healing I desperately need because I don't want it badly enough. You can interpret the Bible however you want, just like any other book—and I find proof that I'm to blame. I wade through parables about not having sufficient faith, disappointed in myself for failing at this, too. My trust in God feels more than adequate. What else can I do?

I word my prayers differently. Instead of casually talking to Jesus after closing my door, I sit up straight in bed, no whispering this time. I put on my most solemn voice and start, "Dear Jesus

Christ of Nazareth," as if using his full name will convince him I am worthy of deliverance. I toy around with praying to God, Jesus, and the Holy Spirit instead of addressing one person, just in case it means my words have a higher chance of making it to the right ears.

I make public declarations to show God that I mean business. My church regularly brings in ministers who talk about the marvelous things they've witnessed. They draw large crowds and high levels of anticipation. Every service ends with an inevitable call to action: Head to the front of the church sanctuary if you need deliverance. They say walking down the aisle is a sign of sacrifice—a way to show your godly devotion to everyone around you.

I take advantage of these opportunities, hoping to have a direct encounter with someone with a special connection to God. I march to the front of the church as gospel music pulses through the sanctuary, trying to ignore the eyes on me, which I may be imagining. I ask God to send these men—they were almost always men—a sign. To let them know that the girl with the glasses who can't stop fidgeting really needs help. To my disappointment, no one ever seems to sense anything. Once, a pastor firmly pushes on my forehead and loudly prays against a spirit of rebellion. I wonder if this is why I am suffering so much. I struggle with the tension of believing that God is all-powerful and my reality. My desperation becomes tangible. *Please, please, please. I promise I believe in you. Please help me.*

I test him by asking for specific, silly signs that he is listening—*God, could you show me three red cars today if you're there?* He disappoints me every time. Meanwhile, my fellow congregants seem to hear so much from him that they can't keep track. In casual conversation, they mention things God has revealed to them or conversations they've had. Preteen me nods along, afraid I'll somehow reveal myself as a fraud if I say too much. A divine being who controls the entire universe and sends unique words to his followers intoxicates me. Hearing from him makes you important. Who wouldn't want that? People pray for things I'm embarrassed to ask for. But they don't care because they wholeheartedly believe the Bible when it says nothing is impossible.

During one church service, the entire congregation gathers around a woman who has an aggressive form of cancer and commands the disease to leave. I join the dozens of people around her and mutter a prayer that she'll be healed, but I don't really believe it. When she dies a few months later, I wonder whether I'm responsible. If God won't do my little miracle—in my opinion, repairing my brain won't take too much effort—I doubt he'll do big ones, either. He's supposedly better than a genie in the sky but doesn't have time for me.

In high school, I become enamored by megachurches with sleek social media presences and young, attractive pastors—a far cry from the small, traditional Black church I attend. I dream of a day I'll fly across the country and visit in person. What the organizations have in common beyond their branding is the emphasis on faith healing. It reignites my desire to trust that God will perform a miracle. I start to read the Bible regularly, taking a highlighter and sparkly gel pen to the pages that stick out to me. Before I begin my homework, I turn on music that sounds like soft rock and sit as still as possible, hoping the quiet creates an environment that God will deem worthy of using for something remarkable.

I am obsessive about how I can make it happen for myself. I keep a prayer journal to document my one-sided conversations with heaven, hoping to eventually learn how to hear him. One day, I wake up with ear pain. I suspect an infection. But I don't tell my parents or ask for antibiotics. Instead, I read Scripture and write prayers in my journal, commanding the ache to leave. Disappointingly, it does not. I seek something impressive to give myself undeniable proof that God is working, but my reality is mundane.

I can't tell you how old I am the first time I speak in tongues, but I know the day is met with fanfare. We believed in receiving the Holy Ghost, and the primary evidence for this spiritual transformation is a heavenly language that sounds like babbling to human ears. Even though God doesn't talk to me, I want something from him. When it is my turn for the gift, I am ready. I repeat "Jesus" over and over, allowing it to become an incoherent chant. It takes a few tries, but I am soon filled with the Spirit. I pray in tongues daily, convinced that healing may be closer if I don't rely on earthly words. Yet again, my strategy fails, and I am no closer to the mental renewal I seek.

I think I was twenty years old the last time I spoke in tongues, but I may have been younger. There's still something about the experience that fascinates me. It is otherworldly to watch someone become so overwhelmed by emotion that they can no longer speak in their native tongue. Sometimes, at church, someone would yell something unintelligible during service, and another person would leap up to translate. Humans can't understand tongues, but God grants the gift of interpretation when he's feeling benevolent.

Pentecostalism is an integral part of my story. When you worship a God who can repair broken limbs and dissolve tumors in milliseconds, all your problems seem manageable. No matter how terrifying, a panic episode is fine because it's temporary suffering. No pain is too immense. I often heard Jesus referred to as "the great physician"—the idea is that he is more effective than any doctor, providing treatment without any need for waiting rooms or co-pays. All you have to do is ask, and he'll heal you. The supernatural wasn't something that shocked us. It was an everyday part of life. The Bible proclaims that signs follow people who believe. We took it at its word.

SEVEN YEARS BEFORE

Finally, I can go home.

The psych ward really isn't that bad. The worst thing is how bored I feel. I'm not traumatized by the experience, but I am ready to leave. On the drive home, I take out my phone—God, I've missed it—and snap a peace sign selfie, my hospital bracelet still on my wrist. I don't know why I take the picture, but I feel like I might want to remember this moment later.

The medication is already working, or maybe that's a placebo effect. All I know is that I'm feeling better than I have in years. My mind drifts to the week prior when I urgently prayed for help. God needed to know that things were heavy—worse than ever. My days hiding my self-inflicted wounds paled in comparison to what I was feeling. If he didn't help, I didn't know what I'd do.

And yet, I feel the same disappointing stillness I've become accustomed to. The car is silent, and no one forces conversation.

I lean my forehead against the cold passenger window, thinking intently. Should God get credit for the past week? Maybe he made sure Dr. Lewis was working during my admission or orchestrated the nursing schedule so I'd get only the kindest ones. I'm being generous. If God was there—and it's a big if—he decided not to heal me, even though the alternative was me wanting to die. He's all-knowing, so this isn't news to him. But he didn't do anything. The devastation I felt at this realization no longer stings as hard. I have other ways to get better now. My desperation morphs into bitterness before I land on cautious acceptance.

I think back to my junior year of high school when I took a monthlong break from social media, opting to spend my idle time praying instead. At one point, I stopped eating lunch with my friends to read my Bible in the empty school library. Was my devotion to God as a teenager genuine or due to my untreated mental health issues? I'm not sure I know the answer—or whether it matters. I think back to my childhood self, secretly suffering from panic attacks and eager for relief. I wonder how much quicker I would have shared my experience with an adult if I weren't raised in a religion that gave me what felt like an out. After all, praying is more accessible than going to a therapist.

I can't decide how I should think about the pleading of my youth. If I look at it with rose-colored glasses, there's something special about my willingness to trust without cynicism. But how much pain could I have been spared if I had gotten professional help sooner? Although I reflect fondly on my childhood, there's little doubt that it would have been even better if I had access to needed resources.

I'm lucky. I didn't experience any long-lasting effects from my time spent praying instead of seeking medical care, which isn't the case for everyone. I was surrounded by people who believed in the validity of medication; if my parents had known how deeply I was suffering, I have no doubt they would've taken me to a psychiatrist. Religious rhetoric can have a profound impact, and I can easily envision a different outcome if I hadn't gotten help for suicidal ideation when I did or my self-harm habit became even more severe. Not everyone makes it out of fundamentalism alive.

I walked away from Pentecostalism and its offshoots in my mid-twenties. Today, I don't spend as much time with people who believe in faith healing, but when I do, the resentful jealousy that once bubbled up inside me is barely there. In years past, hearing someone proclaim the exciting news that God has cured them would've sent me spiraling. That I can be happy for someone for their miracle, real or imagined, is a reality that would've shocked the past me. But even with all my progress, a tiny part of me wonders how different my life would be if God had granted my wish.

I can't explain the allure of a miracle if you didn't grow up wholeheartedly believing, but maybe you get it without my help. Your life changes in an instant. It's like winning the lottery, except the worst parts of your life suddenly disappear instead of receiving a financial windfall. But I have heard plenty about God fixing people's finances, so maybe you get a life upgrade and the money. He's like Santa Claus, but real.

Pentecostalism gave me plenty of fire-and-brimstone preaching about heaven and hell; I was petrified of sinning and ending up eternally damned. God was scary, and I didn't want to make him mad. Our teachings around healing revealed a different side of him—one that I found easier to digest. He wanted the best for me, and that meant he was willing to take away my suffering. I felt conflicted about a God who'd banish people to hell for not worshiping him sufficiently, but a deity who wanted me to feel better was a much easier sell. Plus, everyone loves a bit of mysticism. The idea that you can ease the worst parts of your life by saying a few words is more astonishing than any magic trick.

The question remains: What do you do when it doesn't work? A few years ago, I watched in fascination as a church across the country held a prayer rally to resurrect a child who'd tragically died. The movement spread like wildfire, and there was even a viral hashtag for the cause. Eventually, the prayer rallies stopped, and the family laid the toddler to rest. But how do you come back from that? As far as I can tell, most of the people involved in the services I obsessively live-streamed accepted the death and didn't walk away from the faith because of it. Though thousands of miles away, I felt myself easing into bitterness. Why wouldn't God bring a two-year-old back from the dead if he could? Why not relieve the parents' unimaginable pain? And wouldn't allowing a child to walk out of the coroner's office assuage the doubts of millions of people? I can imagine the headlines now: LOCAL CHILD RAISED FROM THE DEAD! Doubters like me would have no option but to wholeheartedly believe. Right?

If you're religious, you may have responses to the questions I posed. The thing is, I can answer all of them, too. *His ways are higher than ours. We may only have answers once we get to heaven. Sometimes God's idea of healing looks different from what we'd expect.*

I'm not mocking you. If anything, I'm jealous. My skepticism has cost me a lot. People don't come to me for spiritual advice, and I can't blame them, but I have a fair amount of experience trying to make sense of it all.

When I was young, I was so terrified of going to hell that I'd plug my ears when I had a question that seemed like it might be so offensive to God that he'd decide to condemn me. I spent a decade of my life desperately wanting to believe that the God I heard everyone brag about was real. Still, I couldn't reconcile it with my experience. Sure, other folks may talk to him and have their prayers answered, but that clearly wasn't the truth for everyone. Maybe I sinned too much or let my doubts get in the way. Or maybe—and I was afraid to even think it—it's God's fault, not mine.

My upbringing affects how I think of prayer, which is true for all of us. I try to remember that everyone views it differently—some in ways that I find more agreeable. There are actual benefits to prayer, a reality that leaves me feeling equally fascinated and uncomfortable. I stumbled upon a study that found prayer can decrease aggression.[1] Researchers intentionally made the study's participants angry and then asked some of them to pray for someone; those who did reported feeling less mad. For so long, prayer was a shortcut to making *myself* feel better. No wonder I found it futile. I didn't drop to my knees to pray the second I read the research, but it did get me thinking.

The more I learn about the good of prayer, the more tense I feel. For example, the similarities between meditation and prayer are plentiful, which I'd never stopped to consider. There are proven benefits of meditation—it can reduce stress and anxiety, improve focus, help control pain, and more.[2] The same goes for prayer. I love the idea of meditating and don't have conflicting thoughts about it. Meanwhile, talking to God will always be impossibly complicated for me.

Another study examined randomized controlled studies focused on the efficacy of prayer.[3] The studies' results ranged wildly—in some cases, those who prayed or were prayed for seemed to experience better outcomes. In other trials, it made no difference. In at least one study, patients who were prayed for did worse. The researchers conclude that it's difficult to measure the effectiveness of prayer because there are many contributing factors. The discussion section stood out to me.

> If the number, duration, and frequency of prayer are important or if the number of persons praying is important, does God, like a businessman, market boons based on the currency value of the prayers? Or, will God pay attention only if those who pray are sufficiently bothersome?

These questions have bothered me. I haven't publicly asked for prayer in several years, but I've felt comforted in the past when people reached out to share that they were praying during hard times. Despite my complicated relationship with the practice, in the past, I gravitated toward prayer when life got tough, whispering under my breath like a kid again. Call it a supernatural pull, or maybe it's muscle memory. But I still had doubts.

Does having multiple people praying for you make it more likely your prayer will be answered? Will the answer look the same if five people pray for me versus fifty? What if you pray for five minutes versus an hour? Are you more likely to be rewarded if you take the approach I took as a teenager—giving up your favorite things and time with your friends to talk to God? Is there a formula I never cracked?

I still cringe when prayer is offered as the first line of response to mental health conditions—excluding extremists, most people readily accept that a person with diabetes may need insulin or someone with a heart condition could benefit from a pacemaker. The same grace is rarely extended to people who suffer debilitating mental health symptoms. I grew up hearing that I needed to PUSH (Pray Until Something Happens). I pushed with all my might and had little to show for it.

I can torment myself by hunting down the answers I'll never get, or I can make peace with it—that he never gave me what I wanted. I want to settle for the latter. But as hard as I try, I can't shake it completely. What if I *could* make it happen? I dutifully take my antianxiety pills every night but sometimes imagine an alternate universe where God made my problems disappear. The miracle I've been desperate for comes from the prescription I get filled at the pharmacy down the street. I can't imagine anyone at the church of my youth cheering as I yelled that testimony. I force myself to accept it, though—what else can I do?

NINE MONTHS BEFORE

I make my way inside the trendy coffee shop where I'm meeting with an old friend. For once, I am early, which is something of a miracle itself. I pick at my fingernails as I sit and allow myself to daydream. I no longer ruminate on the mystery of the supernatural, and I've accepted that God can be found in less tangible ways. I feel him when I laugh until my stomach hurts when I'm with good friends and a bottle of wine or when my husband and I play board games and each lets the other win as we learn to fall in love all over again. The divine feels clearest when I'm on a plane to an unfamiliar destination, ready to explore the world, or snuggled up in bed with my favorite book.

I don't need to speak in tongues or read the Bible daily. I could be spiritual without being relentlessly devout. Life isn't what I'd envisioned, but it is still worth living. I don't have all the answers—far from it, actually—but I am content.

In less than a year, I'll become God's chosen prophet.

CHAPTER THREE

Raising Hell

Ayana is struggling to tell the difference between delusions and reality.
—My Clinical Documentation Record, page 198

THREE YEARS BEFORE

We wandered into a bar on a sticky summer night, looking for a cozy place to end the evening. The drinks were expensive but surprisingly delicious, the perfect mix of liquor and fruit. I took a picture of my smiling date to capture the moment—string lights in the background and cocktail glasses beaded with condensation on the table.

Then, I made the mistake of sharing it on social media.

The Wednesday after that bar visit, I sat at my desk at the trendy marketing agency where I worked, bland pop music playing faintly in the background. I glanced at my lit-up phone and saw my husband's name on the screen. It was unusual for him to reach out during the workday, so I sped to the office lobby before picking up.

His manager had seen the picture I posted and called him into a meeting in his office to discuss it. My husband and his boss were very different, but they had something in common. They both made a living playing music at one of the biggest churches in the city. My husband was told he wasn't in trouble. (Naturally, this was a sign he might be in trouble.) His boss was concerned about my motive for posting alcoholic drinks publicly. My husband was furious; this wasn't the first time he felt his manager had overstepped.

As he relayed this, I felt impossibly small and wanted to sink into the sidewalk outside the office building. I had made a colossal mistake. Of course my actions impacted him. Was it worth risking his career so I could fire off a tweet for a few likes? Why hadn't I thought about how it could turn out? The rationale his manager gave was that my post could cause someone to drink, leading to a lapse in judgment. Or maybe someone who'd had a partying habit would find themselves drawn back to the lifestyle. His boss asked my husband if he'd stopped to think how my behavior would reflect on him.

Frustration took over. "I. Don't. Work. There!" I nearly yelled. We ended the conversation, and I fought back tears as I returned to my computer. I'd messed up. I'd had no reservations at the time, but now I realized that I should not have shared the photo.

I loved my job, and I loved that it wasn't at the building where my husband stood on stage every Sunday as a worship leader. They held him to rules that I had little interest in following; meanwhile, my coworkers talked freely, and there were office happy hours that you could post on social media without any repercussions. But the people at the church viewed me as an extension of my husband and held me to the same code of conduct that he had to follow, even though I hadn't signed up for it. No one said it aloud, but they didn't have to. I'd attended enough churches to know how it worked.

I have a target on my back, I thought. I'm sick of this.

My eyelids are heavy, which is a rarity lately. Sleep and I are no longer friends. But the voice jolts me, and it is time for another word from God. This one is a doozy. We're going to start a church. My husband and I. I can't wait to tell him.

It will be the biggest church in the world, and everyone who comes will help spread the word about my book. That's one of the ways it's going to become a bestseller. The other ways haven't been revealed to me yet. What's in this book, anyway? He'll tell me eventually, I hope. He has to. It hasn't been long since he started talking, but I already trust him more than anyone I know.

I am wide awake as he fills me in on the details. No building in the world is big enough to hold us, so we settle for stadiums and arenas. People line up outside Madison Square Garden and wait for hours, hoping to snag a seat at our packed services. Our events are broadcast on international news channels—no one can get enough. And the best part? Everyone loves me so much that I don't have to change anything about myself. I can drink and say the occasional curse word, and no one will care. I finally won't feel self-conscious anymore. It's what I've always wanted.

Meanwhile, everyone we know will move to us to help us launch. We'll be surrounded by all our loved ones, even those who aren't religious. They won't be able to resist, just like I'm not. I digest all he's saying and try to process it. A couple of years ago, I would've recoiled at the idea. Honestly, I'm not sure how to feel. It sounds like a lot of work for someone with dwindling faith in organized religion. I don't want to be a pastor.

But he doesn't make mistakes, so I need to listen.

ELEVEN YEARS BEFORE

I spotted an unfamiliar boy when I walked into my best friend's kitchen. He had a quiet voice and brown hair that flopped in his face. After he introduced himself, I found myself looking for a second too long. He wasn't my type—can you have a type at fifteen?—but I was drawn to him. We talked, and he invited me to his church. When Sunday night arrived, I watched in awe as he strummed his guitar at the front of the small building. We sang Hillsong choruses in hushed tones. The person next to me was crying. The maybe-crush quickly blossomed. Sure, he was a little cute, but he was also anointed by God.

I began to picture our lives together. Being married to a church musician—or a worship leader, as we called them—was a thrilling thought. I thought of myself in the front row, swaying to the music as my husband sang. Everyone would be jealous that I'd landed him. In one of our first conversations on AOL Instant Messenger, he told me that a prophet once told him his musical talents would get him far one day. Since then, he'd known he had a gift. I was jealous that I hadn't received divine instruction about my future.

Two years after we met, he asked me to be his girlfriend. At the time, it was the best day of my life. Three years later, he took me on a walk and got down on one knee with a ring I'd picked, a photographer hiding in the bushes. Our lives were coming together. Then, he aced the first interview at a megachurch—a behemoth organization with roughly twenty thousand parishioners. The wedding was only a few months away, and everything was falling into place. We'd relocate for his dream job, and I'd find something I loved, too.

I had some reservations about his career. My father started a church when I was thirteen years old, and I'll never forget the amount of scrutiny I felt as a member of the pastor's family. I don't know if the attention was imagined, but the anxiety was present nonetheless. We had no choice but to be involved—teaching children about the Bible, showing up to outreach events, and even singing in front of the congregation (off-key, in my case) when there were no other options. The rest of my family enjoyed it, but I struggled. I told God I wouldn't ever marry a pastor.

I guess my prayer wasn't specific enough, because my husband's new job meant I'd still face unwanted attention. He wasn't leading a church, but some of the same rules applied. No more sneaking into service late or skipping Sundays because I needed the rest. We were a unit, and that meant I had to be spiritually devout, too. I started to read my Bible more to prepare. Messing it up was the last thing I wanted.

The first months after the move were a whirlwind. I made friends quickly and always had a full social calendar. We attended service multiple times a month, and I always picked a seat near the front, dutiful wife that I was. I was living out my teenage dream of being married to someone special, and it was even more exciting than I had imagined. But things took a turn as the 2016 election season ramped up, and I saw the church become tacitly political. I started to feel self-conscious about my views, which were to the left of nearly all my friends there.

Was it paranoia? I told myself I was probably imagining things, but it became clear that some people didn't seem to like me very much, which was a painful truth for a chronic people pleaser. Modern Christianity has many faults, and I felt a call to speak up about them—on social media, in written articles, and face-to-face. That came at a cost. My desire to be well-received fell flat. In my last conversation with my husband's boss, he told us he'd consciously chosen not to "pursue a relationship" with us. I couldn't help but feel that my straightforwardness—my tweets expressing disappointment in how the church treats undocumented immigrants and my email to the lead pastor after someone said something markedly offensive—ruined everything. This reality devastated me. Wanting to be loved is a hell of a drug.

My honesty came at a steep cost, but was the punishment deserved? In an environment where capitulation is expected, and men are the only ones allowed to be aggressive, my frankness wasn't a fit, even though my behavior was arguably not that problematic. Some lessons are learned only by living them. And I couldn't help but remember teenage Ayana who had no desire to be involved in church ministry as an adult. She may have been onto something.

I want you to know that not every moment from that time was terrible. Our apartment often burst at the seams with friends we loved, people we still care for years later. It is all painfully complicated, the duality of birthday parties, weekend trips, vibrant group chats, and some of the hardest things we've lived.

The microaggressions were brutal.

One time, my husband sat in the back seat of a car while one of the church's musicians drove. As the man weaved in and out of traffic, he jokingly spat out the N-word—hard *r* and all, assuming my husband, a fellow White man, would be okay with it. My husband expressed his disgust to the man; the coworker wrote him an apology letter. But it's hard to go back to small talk once you've seen someone at their nastiest.

A couple of months later, I swiveled in my husband's office chair, waiting for him to meet me for lunch. Then, I heard an all-too-loud conversation outside his door. A White church official was mocking how Black people spoke, putting on a stereotypical Blaccent for giggles. The other people in the conversation laughed loudly. I waited for them to leave before I snuck out, crying silently. I wasn't hungry anymore. When my husband confronted the issue, he was told that comedian Dave Chappelle makes fun of White people. What's the difference?

This isn't the first time I'd experienced subtle prejudice.

Somehow, my parents have kept all my class photos stacked in boxes in the garage. I was one of twenty-three students in my kindergarten picture, but the only one with a brown face. Later, some of my elementary school classmates decided Ayana was too hard to pronounce. "Can we call you Kiera?" they asked. I was confused but desperate to fit in, as all kids are, so I said yes. I responded to my new moniker with pride. I later learned that Kiera was a Black girl who had previously attended the school. Although the

Pentecostal church of my youth was wonderfully diverse and gave me friends who looked like me, the dozens of hours spent at school every week had an impact. I started to resent my bigger lips and wide hips, wishing I looked more like my White classmates. In high school, several of my fellow students casually used racial slurs around me. I smiled as if being degraded would make them like me more. It did, and it does.

THREE MONTHS BEFORE

The news anchor gave a solemn warning about potentially disturbing content ahead. Then, the screen was filled with an image so horrific that I attempted to plug my ears and cover my eyes at the same time. His name was George Floyd, and I couldn't escape the video of his murder. I had no choice but to watch, to stand witness to the brutality of racism.

I didn't know what to do. I scrolled on my phone in an attempt to briefly distract myself from the violence, but it was everywhere I looked. The moment's impact encouraged me—rage seemed to fill everyone around me, even the apolitical ones—but I still felt helpless. I had to say something. I opened Instagram and posted a video about the importance of non-Black people speaking out. Suddenly, the post went viral. My views skyrocketed, and I gained nearly forty thousand followers in a week.

I was invited to podcasts and news programs to discuss systemic racism and Black health disparities. Advocating in this way was all I'd ever wanted, but a part of me felt shame for being too loud, too divisive, too abrasive. I knew I wouldn't get in trouble for my words—I was self-employed, and by this point, we attended a progressive church that didn't think God wanted everyone to vote Republican. After my husband quit the megachurch job, I wrote about the things that mattered to me without worrying about retribution. And I could have a margarita in public without any fear it would trigger a meeting. But the humiliation I'd felt when I learned he was in hot water at work because of something I did was hard to shake. Part of me still thought I'd ruined his dream; although he maintained that he was ready to leave the church, I knew the drama I'd inadvertently caused played a part in his decision. I was freer than ever, but it didn't matter.

Some version of me still believed there was a specific formula that a Good Wife followed. She is subservient, yielding to her husband without complaint. A social media rant is far beneath her; if she has any strong opinions, she doesn't feel the need to share them with the world. The Good Wife effortlessly whips up homemade bread whenever people come over (boiling pasta is the extent of my culinary prowess). She is also irritatingly beautiful, someone who somehow looks better without makeup. Most importantly, she doesn't flip any tables.

It didn't matter that my husband insisted he wanted the most authentic version of me, not an unrealistic standard I'd created in my head. Nor did I care that thousands of people were cheering me on. I still felt naked every time I hit "post," even if it was something innocuous. A friend had once received a rebuke from another parishioner for posting a picture of herself in a bathing suit. Ignorance wasn't an excuse. The tension between who I was and who I thought I should be was all-consuming. Being my husband's wife was no longer my most important title, but I couldn't escape the pressure I'd put on myself.

I took a selfie weeks before our wedding, before moving my belongings to our new place. I look unbelievably young, and my smile is so big that it stretches my features. The difference is stark from when I left our apartment a few miles from the megachurch for the last time—jaded, hurt, and wary. This time, I was only happy because I was leaving.

After moving on from the megachurch, I reached a comfortable place. Although I no longer pleaded with God to perform miracles, he still fascinated me. I read the Bible most mornings to satisfy my curiosity and counted down to church services, excited to jot notes during the sermon. But things started to change. I realized my nonreligious manager treated me kindlier than some of the people I dealt with at church; my coworkers were more inclusive than any prayer group I'd joined. I didn't know everything about Jesus, but it started to feel like he'd fit in better at happy hour than among those in pews every Sunday.

I started to wonder why I was a Christian in the first place. The faith that once excited me suddenly looked dull. I didn't want to spend time with people who believed my friends would go to hell for who they loved. Explaining human rights to fellow churchgoers, hoping they'd view me as worthy, was no longer acceptable. I was over it. Done with begging people to recognize my humanity. Tired of spending my time worshiping next to people with bigoted beliefs. It was no longer meant for me. I couldn't believe I'd ever been okay with my husband's old job. Attending church felt like a stretch. How did I ever think he could've worked at one without it blowing up in our faces? My husband started to play guitar a couple of times a month at our new church, and even that felt like too much. Being behind the scenes for so long gave me a unique, terrible perspective. It's like going into a restaurant's kitchen, seeing cockroaches, and returning to the table to finish your meal. Easier said than done, right? I was perfectly happy to be someone who visited church infrequently, blissfully unaware of the dysfunction happening out of sight.

Teenage me was fiercely envious of my husband and his gift, jealous that I hadn't received divine instruction about my future. But I can now see the implications of telling a child they have a magnificent calling that'll change people's lives. How could that not create immense pressure—from family members, fellow churchgoers, and yourself—to live up to the message you've received? Unabashedly daydreaming about the future is one of the purest things about childhood. When I was in elementary school, I wanted to be an actor, then a model, then a scientist because—and I quote an old homework assignment—I'd heard they made fifty dollars an hour. I cycled through these possibilities, free to dream about my options without a revelatory word in the back of my head. Knowing your eventual path when you aren't old enough to do long division feels, ironically enough, uninspired.

I couldn't remember the last time I read my Bible, and I sometimes closed my eyes and pretended when people asked me to pray. I realized that many of the divine prophetic words I'd heard in church were no more specific than the daily astrology readings I sometimes looked up out of curiosity. *God had a great plan for me, and I would do something incredible for him one day.* Big surprise.

My ties to Pentecostalism were gone, which part of me mourned, but I was no longer bound by religion. The fervent Christianity of my childhood was now foreign, but I was more assured than ever, more than when I sang songs every Sunday or taught lessons as a youth group leader. I felt more confident than I'd been at my most devout, when I wanted to save my non-Christian friends from burning for eternity. The beliefs I settled on would be considered blasphemous by many, but they were all right for me. As my faith and politics shifted, I unlearned things I'd believed my entire life. It was terrifying yet exhilarating.

I was content until I was no longer in control—then I became ravenous for answers from God. When psychosis came rushing in, I proclaimed the good news about Jesus to anyone who would listen. Suddenly, it felt impossible to remain silent, no matter what my outspokenness might cost me.

I am in heaven, and it is even better than I imagined.

God brought me up here when I started to ask too many questions. "I'm so sorry," I say, but he just laughs.

"It's okay," he responds.

The light is so bright that I struggle to fully open my eyes. When I do, I'm greeted by a vision so powerful it nearly knocks me down. I am seeing God for the first time. He is too much to describe. I'd put him into words if I could, but I don't have any. I wish I had a notebook to draw what he's showing me, but my hands are empty. I'll commit it all to memory. When we start the church, I'll tell everyone about this trip. It's one of the reasons we draw huge crowds. I've spent much time thinking about heaven—first, terrified of not making it, then pondering if it's even real—so this is a crucial moment. I have the proof I've always needed. Wait. This is what the book is about! Maybe.

I shouldn't get ahead of myself.

I feel confused as I look around. Heaven isn't as impressive as I thought it'd be. There are no golden streets or pearly gates. But what I can see is even more stunning. People of all ages, genders, and ethnicities walk hand in hand. It's not like a college admissions brochure aiming to tick off diversity boxes. You can tell they're all delightfully comfortable with themselves. It is the most beautiful thing I've ever seen.

Why can't my life be like this? I've wasted twenty-seven years desperately trying to shrink into spaces that weren't meant for me. I've spent my existence afraid. Wary of what others think when they look at me. Stressed that ultrareligious people are mad about my opinions. Scared of the way my skin color will affect me. Everything I've been told is a beautiful lie. None of it matters. I don't want to go back to Earth, but I have to start the church.

We're going to change the world.

CHAPTER FOUR

The Worst Day

She needs constant reassurance that she is safe.
—My Clinical Documentation Record, page 151

SIXTEEN MONTHS BEFORE

The video is just over a minute long and filmed in a Walgreens parking lot. The smile on my face is so big that it's nearly cartoonish. "I'm . . . pregnant?" I tell the camera before covering my mouth in disbelief. I am at the pharmacy to buy another pregnancy test. The two I took at home that morning were decidedly positive, but I still couldn't believe it. I immediately called my ob-gyn's office and froze when they asked why I needed to come in, afraid that if I said it aloud, it'd disappear like a mirage. "I feel like I'm dreaming, and this isn't real," I confide into my phone. "Stay tuned."

My husband has plans to hang out with friends after work; I call him and say I don't feel well to get him to come straight home. I am practically bursting with the news and devise a creative way to share. I tuck the pregnancy tests in a bathroom drawer and covertly film his reaction. He gingerly holds a test, not caring that I'd recently dipped it in urine. The end of the video is shakier than a clip from *The Blair Witch Project* as I rush to embrace him. We are going to have a baby.

I drive the twenty minutes to my parents' house to tell them. I know most people wait to reveal their pregnancies, but it feels like news too good to keep to myself. My head starts to spin, thinking about the future. We'll have to turn the office into a nursery and figure out what to do for childcare. I think about our finances and whether we are ready. Should we have waited? I brush off my mounting worries to enjoy what is supposed to be the best day of my life. An online calculator tells me the baby is due in December. The best Christmas gift. I start to feel better.

As a child, I didn't aspire to motherhood—I know people who dreamed about their families from when they were old enough to play with dolls, but I'm not one of them. Part of me plans to have kids because that is what you are supposed to do once you reach a certain age; my career has always excited me more than a hypothetical family. A couple of years into marriage, the idea became more appealing. My friends started to have babies, and I pictured my future as I oohed and aahed over their children. I knew it was a matter of when, not if, and my husband felt the same.

We took a grand trip to Europe as one last hurrah before trying to conceive, hunting for cheap flight deals and dipping into our joint savings account to cover our adventure. As we got selfies in front of the Eiffel Tower and saw the sights in London, I wondered whether I'd miss the independence that comes when no one depends on you for survival. But I felt excited, picturing myself cradling my swollen belly and comparing diaper brands. Life will soon change drastically, but it'll be for the better.

As I battle all the intense, conflicting emotions that can come after a positive pregnancy test, I thought about my work. I'd quit my corporate job and taken a leap to full-time freelancing only six weeks prior. My client list isn't very long, and there isn't anyone offering to pay for my maternity leave. Crunching the numbers makes me think that things will be tight for a while. I'm only twenty-five years old; my psychiatrist didn't have her first child till she was in her early forties. I shake these thoughts, feeling guilty that I'm experiencing anything other than pure joy.

The early weeks are filled with the excitement of a first pregnancy. I surprise all my family members and friends with the news, capturing their shocked faces for a compilation video I later put on YouTube. Pictures from ultrasound appointments fill my camera roll—me trying to keep up as the sonographer describes what I am looking at. I subsist on crackers and ginger candy when the nausea becomes too much to bear.

After dinner with my family one night, I get sick in a parking lot, which sends my husband back into the restaurant to grab handfuls of napkins so I can clean myself up. "One day, I'll make our baby feel bad for doing this to me," I joke. The first trimester is far from glamorous, but I feel myself adjusting to a new rhythm. Naps become regular, and I exercise sporadically. Sometimes, willing myself to walk our dog halfway down the block is the extent of my physical activity.

I know my pregnancy might not be perfect—bad things happen to good people all the time. But when I think about an unexpected twist, it is always something surmountable: developing gestational diabetes or high blood pressure, for example. Miscarriage isn't on my mind. Fate can be hopelessly callous, but I have no reason to think it will ever happen to me.

I gather my things, ready to leave the exam room, when a nurse enters. "The doctor wants to have a word with you," she says. It feels akin to being called to the principal's office. I don't know what's happening, but I know it isn't good. The doctor is a nice enough man in his forties, but he's always no-nonsense in our interactions. Before, I questioned his bedside manner, but now I'm glad there's no sugarcoating. We sit in his office, and he looks me in the eye. I sit and nod as he talks, willing myself not to cry.

He doesn't want to create unnecessary panic, he tells me, but the ultrasound technician flagged a potential concern from the scan I had just minutes before. There might be tissue developing outside of the baby's skull. It could be nothing, or it could mean the fetus is incompatible with life.

Incompatible. With. Life. I mouth the words to myself, willing them to sink in. Moments prior, I'd taken a video of the large screen mounted on the wall and watched in wonder as the baby moved its tiny limbs. I wasn't looking at a blob anymore. I've never seen anyone more alive than my baby. And now I know we might never meet. Everything else becomes a blur. *We want to refer you . . . urgent consult . . . high-risk . . . better idea of what's happening.* I thank the doctor for his time and mercifully make it to the lobby before breaking down.

Maybe you've also had a doctor look at you with sympathetic eyes while letting you know that your life might fall apart—or it could be nothing! I don't know how to reconcile the two possibilities as I weigh them. It's probably a fluke. How could it not be? But what if it's real, and the baby is seriously hurt? When I peer at the sonogram I'm given, I think I can see something near the baby's head. If the doctor hadn't just explained the potential severity of the situation, I would've brushed it off. But now, there's no denying it. I call the number I've been given and schedule an appointment for the following week. Now, I have no choice but to wait.

I refer to this time as the Week of Uncertainty, but that's only true in retrospect—I start to feel pretty sure nothing is wrong. I talk to a friend who received a terrifying diagnosis while pregnant. Her child is now a healthy teenager with no medical issues. Doctors get things wrong all the time, I reassure myself. I travel across the state to speak at a networking event and talk confidently about my pregnancy to the crowd.

Most people in my life have no clue that something might be wrong, which I prefer. I don't need sympathetic looks from loved ones when dealing with a nothingburger. Father's Day comes four days after my doctor's appointment. I buy my husband a newborn-sized soccer jersey and a card describing what a great father he'll soon be. We'll get the high-risk visit out of the way and return to normal life.

An estimated 10–20 percent of pregnancies end in loss, but that number may be as high as 30 percent.[1] You likely know someone who has had a miscarriage, whether they've told you or not. There's a reason to remain silent—research shows pregnancy loss is often viewed as taboo by sufferers. Nearly half of those who've experienced miscarriages feel guilty, and 28 percent feel ashamed.[2]

Genetic abnormalities cause most miscarriages and cannot be prevented.[3] Although some risk factors potentially make loss more likely—hormonal conditions, uncontrolled diabetes, and uterine issues—chromosomal problems are to blame for the vast majority of losses.[4] However, misconceptions about pregnancy loss abound. One study found that 76 percent of people think stress can cause miscarriages, and more than 60 percent say lifting a heavy object could induce one. The lack of comprehensive education about pregnancy loss, its frequency, and its causes is a disservice to everyone, whether they've experienced a miscarriage or not.

It can take a severe mental and physical toll. Along with the intense grief that can surround the experience, the body responds viscerally; some experience contractions akin to the pain of childbirth while waiting for their pregnancies to pass. It's not uncommon to feel alone after pregnancy loss, even with a robust support system.

I know none of these statistics. I have a couple friends who suffered miscarriages, and I mainly avoid the topic when talking to them. Terrified of saying the wrong thing, I opt for silence instead of support. During one anxious night early in pregnancy, I google the risk of miscarriage and find a website that spits out data after you share how far along you are. The probability decreases daily, which eases my mind. At eight weeks pregnant, my chances of a viable pregnancy are more than 94 percent. Anyone would like those odds.

FIFTEEN MONTHS BEFORE

I am wearing a blue floral dress rented for the occasion. My husband sits on the kitchen counter behind me with his hands on my stomach. In my hand, I hold a sonogram. We are smiling. The professional photographer does her job well—we look effortlessly good.

I impatiently wait for her to email me the photos. When she does, I leap into action and carefully type out the caption. "Christmas is gonna be real special this year . . . because I'm PREGNANT!" I open Instagram. I tap the share button. On Facebook, I take a different approach: "Santa isn't the only one coming to town this Christmas!" I am proud of my cleverness.

I refresh both apps incessantly to watch the likes flood in. People use social media to help them feel less alone. To document their lives. To connect with long-lost friends. I keep up with my accounts for these reasons, too. But the dopamine hit that comes when the algorithmic gods smile down and a post does well is unbeatable. This isn't comfortable to admit. I can only hope I'm not the only one.

I get thousands of likes and hundreds of comments. This is the part I've been eagerly awaiting—sharing our happy news with the world. The response is even better than I imagined. Congratulatory text messages overload my phone. I begin to think about how I'll document my pregnancy online. I'll share an essay online about finding out and keeping it a secret. Maybe a nursery inspiration post after that?

I sometimes quip that I love attention, but it's not entirely a joke. I started a blog when I was twenty-four years old, and I've developed a modest social media following over the years. You only publicly chronicle every aspect of daily life if you are okay with people looking at you. Am I so eager to share my pregnancy because it gives me content for the internet? If I were a more private person, would I wait? But the people around me—family, friends, acquaintances, perfect strangers—are thrilled. I know the baby will be loved.

FOURTEEN MONTHS BEFORE

Ayana wakes up and throws on an oversized sweatshirt emblazoned with the mascot of her alma mater, even though it is summertime. She is too distracted to care that it's hot—today, she will finally get the reassurance she's been waiting for all week. Ayana invites her parents to join her at the appointment. She later wonders whether she'd sensed it deep down.

She goes to Starbucks and orders a sausage-and-egg breakfast sandwich, no cheese. Google Maps says she'll arrive on time. Ayana is usually late, so she feels proud of herself. She sits down in the waiting room and allows her mind to wander. Maybe there is something serious going on, like a brain injury. She brushes off the thought.

The ultrasound room barely fits her and her husband, let alone her parents. Still, she is surrounded by the people she loves most, and they'll all look at her baby together. The ultrasound jelly is warm. An image flashes across the screen. The baby isn't moving like it did last time. The sonographer doesn't say anything. Ayana prefers it when they're friendly, pointing out the baby's features and letting her record the *woosh-woosh-woosh* of the heartbeat, but maybe this sonographer is having a bad day.

The technician excuses herself, and Ayana hops off the exam table to clean herself up. The jelly always gets everywhere. She hopes it won't stain her pants. This is the worst part of her day so far.

The doctor enters the room. She has sad eyes. Why does she look like that? Before Ayana can spiral at the possibilities, the obstetrician opens her mouth. *No heartbeat I'm sorry rare birth defect genetic counselor I am so, so sorry.* Ayana yells, "No no no no NO." On a typical day, this would embarrass her. She hates making a scene. Today, she wishes to scream even louder—she wants everyone in the building to hear.

Then, there's the genetic counselor. Ayana wonders what being on call for people's worst moments is like. She hopes the nice woman sitting in front of her is paid well. She says words Ayana has never heard before. "We can conduct a fetal autopsy," the counselor says. "We can offer genetic testing for you and your husband for future children."

"Okay," Ayana responds. "Okay."

She's never considered what happens when your body betrays you and you're no longer carrying a fetus with a heartbeat. She feels like a walking cemetery. The nice doctor tells her to call her ob-gyn to discuss her next steps. Ayana doesn't remember whether her husband made the call or her parents. She has no idea what it feels like to walk out of an office filled with visibly pregnant patients. She will forget the thirty-minute drive from the high-risk center to her regular doctor. But the rest of the day sticks with her.

The receptionist asks what time her appointment is; Ayana starts sobbing. "I am here," she chokes out, "because I am having a miscarriage." The woman's face changes; her voice softens. Ayana is ushered into an exam room where a nurse explains her options. She can wait for the pregnancy to pass at home or opt for surgery to remove the fetal tissue. "Whatever is fastest, please," Ayana says like she's ordering at a restaurant in a rush. The doctor—the same one who first told her last week something might be wrong—recommends the surgery.

"Okay," she says. "Okay."

She goes to the emergency room and is transferred to the hospital's pre-op area. She changes into a hospital gown. Ayana realizes she hasn't asked her husband how he's doing. Her grief is so all-consuming that it feels like it may swallow her whole.

The following hours are full of waiting, waiting, waiting. Finally, they explain the surgery to her. The doctor will use a special tool to scrape her uterine lining and remove everything. She stops herself from interjecting that *everything* is her baby. Ayana will be put under sedation and sleep through the whole thing. This part is a relief. She signs consent forms; a nurse tells her the procedure will happen later than planned.

Finally, it is time. The anesthesiologist tells her she must remove her nose ring; she asks him to tape it instead. Today is hard enough without wrestling the tiny hoop out of her face. He agrees. She wonders if he feels bad for her. Ayana says goodbye to her husband as they wheel her to the operating room. She cannot bring herself to say goodbye to the baby. She will soon drift off to sleep. When she wakes up, she will no longer be pregnant.

She is me, and I am her, but it all happened to someone else. I later learned this is a coping mechanism.

You have a 1-in-10,000 chance of finding a four-leaf clover, according to a webpage with so many pop-ups that it probably infected my laptop with malware.

You have a 1-in-10,400 chance of birthing a child with an encephalocele, a clunky word that stumped me the first time I tried to spell it. If you are the Centers for Disease Control and Prevention, an encephalocele is "a sac-like protrusion of the brain and membranes that cover it through an opening in the skull."[5] If you are me, it is the reason I lost my baby.

I am desperate to know what I should have done differently. Some days, I was too nauseous to take my prenatal vitamin, even though I knew it was essential for a baby's development. I'd only craved fried foods and turned my nose up at salads. And I sometimes felt conflicted about the baby and whether we were ready—maybe this is a form of cosmic punishment. I'd gotten pregnant easily, but did I deserve a baby?

I took an antidepressant during my pregnancy. I accepted the risks because the benefits seemed to outweigh them. The genetic counselor assures me that the medication that saved my life didn't cause the defect to develop. Later, while writing, I stumbled upon a study released after my miscarriage that found a link between antidepressant use in pregnancy and an increased chance of congenital abnormalities.[6] I closed my browser and tried to pretend I didn't see it. I had a one-in-three chance of miscarrying the week I found out I was pregnant. The day I lost the baby, the probability of miscarriage was 1.3 percent. I'd let my guard down because the chance was practically zero. It is one of my biggest regrets.

As a child, I regularly felt terror overtake me as I realized with certainty that I was going to die that night. I'd lie in bed and repent for all the sins I'd committed to make sure I didn't go to hell when I passed. When I couldn't think of any carnal mistakes I'd made, I'd ask God to forgive any evil I'd done and subsequently forgotten about. On some level, I knew the fear was too irrational to share with anyone else. I would never give my parents a teary goodbye or tell my friends I'd never see them again. And I grasped that the chance I'd randomly die in my sleep was probably low.

When I wasn't contemplating my impending death, I pictured awful things happening to the people I love. These weren't unwelcome thoughts—I willed myself to conjure up car crashes, fires, shootings, and cancer diagnoses. What were the chances I would imagine my father being injured in an accident on his way home from work and it would actually occur? To save the people I loved, I had to visualize them dying in horrific, gruesome ways. I became obsessed with all the unfortunate yet unavoidable tragedies that can happen to someone. I still sometimes find myself lost in thought about all the dreadful things that might happen to my family.

I can't help but resent my therapist after the miscarriage. If I'd allowed myself to focus on every possibility the way I had years ago—if I hadn't internalized every tool and homework assignment she'd given me—I could have reversed the result. I envision myself researching the worst and repeating sentences to myself. *I will have a baby with a rare birth defect. My pregnancy will not make it.* It's the opposite of a regular affirmation. Instead of putting words into the universe hoping they'll come true, I say my worst-case scenarios aloud to ensure they remain false.

If I can't find a cause for the miscarriage, I'll blame positive thinking.

I am hit with a nauseating realization as I lie in the hospital bed waiting for surgery preparation to begin, the dead fetus inside my body: Everyone knows I'm pregnant. I've even told our next-door neighbors. I think about celebrities who share cryptic Instagram posts to announce their divorces. "This is an amicable decision," they say. I've pitied them for feeling like they owed us their most painful moments. How do you tell the world about something so raw? The pain belongs to me. It is my husband's, too, but I am not ready to share it. I do not want condolences from college professors and childhood friends. And yet.

The white roses sit in a vase on the floor of our living room. In front of the flowers are two sonogram pictures, the last glimpses of my baby. My hand is barely in the frame. I kneel to take the picture. The caption begins, "There's no easy way to share this." The likes and comments roll in just like they did weeks earlier. This time, I do not excitedly check my phone.

The gifts arrive immediately and continue for weeks. Flowers, wind chimes, food delivery gift cards, plants, figurines, books, sentimental jewelry. The companies I freelance for tell me to take all the time I need. My house is filled with concerned friends and family members. "We are cared for," I tell myself. It is a comfort.

When I announce my miscarriage, I'm still wearing heavy-duty pads to absorb the bleeding and contorting myself when a cramp hits. My body and soul are anguished. I sob in bed. It is too soon to share this information with the world. But once I start to talk, something breaks. People are grateful. My inbox is filled with people thanking me for my honesty. "I had a miscarriage, too," they write. I begin to feel better. My first blog post after the miscarriage is full of too much information. Still, I honor the need I felt to share it all. My hurt is so deep-rooted that I want everyone to feel it with me. I write and write and write.

A few months later, an editor from my former workplace asks whether I'd draft an essay on my experience. I jump at the opportunity. When the photographer comes to take pictures for the article, I start crying. I am mortified, but he reassures me that it's okay. In the photos, my husband and I stare somberly at the camera. The piece runs in the newspaper on a Sunday in October. The headline reads, I LOST MY BABY. IT SHOULDN'T BE A SECRET. I am flooded with emails and comments from people who understand my pain.

I expected to spend the summer exhausting delivery workers with package after package of tiny clothes and themed furniture for the baby's room. Instead, our mailbox overflows with medical bills. It seems like everyone wants a piece. My obstetrician, the anesthesiologist, the laboratory where the inconclusive fetal autopsy was conducted—it is equal parts overwhelming and infuriating. I would have happily paid labor and delivery medical bills, but this is unfair.

Nearly a month after my surgery, I see an email with the subject line, "Your results are ready." I opted for the genetic test while eleven weeks pregnant, excited for it to tell me the sex of the baby. I didn't pay attention to all the medical conditions it tested for. I stare at my computer screen. It reads: "POSITIVE FOR TRISOMY 18" in bright red letters. The disorder happens when a baby has an extra copy of the eighteenth chromosome. It is likely responsible for the development of the encephalocele. This will all matter to me eventually. But all I can see is the word next to the diagnosis. *Male*. We would've had a boy. I call my husband, inconsolable. The pain is too much.

I must try to get better, so I reach a conclusion. The only way to move past the miscarriage is by trusting I've had my life's share of bad luck. Things won't be perfect, but I won't be ill-fated. I no longer have to worry about my family members dying in car accidents. Surely God, or the universe, will recognize that I've suffered enough. If anything this bad happens again, I'm not sure what I'll do. And I won't know how to survive if I find myself on the wrong side of the odds again.

Postpartum psychosis occurs in 1 to 2 per 1,000 births.

The baby isn't real.

I sink to the ground. God keeps surprising me, but this one isn't possible. The ultrasound appointments are vivid in my memory. What do you mean? I don't dare mouth the question, even though they're making me wear a surgical mask, and no one can see my lips move. I don't want my enemies to know he talks to me.

He repeats himself, louder this time. The baby wasn't real. The miscarriage was fake. Even if you'd stayed pregnant, no baby would've been born. It was all a test from me to see if you could make it. You passed.

He usually fills me with wonder, but this time, I am speechless. Losing the baby ruined me. Left me a shell of myself. I still dream about what could've been. And it was all a game?

For a short, terrible moment, I doubt his voice. Why would he do that?

CHAPTER FIVE

A Mother's Love

Patient arrived voluntarily. She wants help.
—My Clinical Documentation Record, page 83

NINE MONTHS BEFORE

I scroll through Airbnb until a listing catches my eye: a modest guest suite in North Carolina, only fifteen minutes from downtown Asheville. I swipe through pictures of a cozy fireplace and spacious bedroom. When I look out the window, I'll see mountains. It is perfect.

I've always loved Christmas—the festive lights, corny music, and brainstorming gifts for the people I love. But this year is different. My baby was due days before Christmas, but there will be no celebrating. Everyone else seems to have moved on from the miscarriage, but I am stuck. The unfairness of the situation still overwhelms me, and the idea of a happy holiday at home feels laughable. I jumped at the idea when my husband suggested an end-of-year trip. I book the rental and work on our itinerary; soon, we have plans to visit breweries, trendy food spots, and local coffee shops. My sadness morphs into excitement as our vacation grows closer.

I toss thick sweaters and tall boots into my suitcase, excited for the change in weather. When I go to the bathroom to grab my toiletry bag, I see the pregnancy tests I keep under the sink. I pause. Getting back on birth control after the loss didn't appeal to me—I still wanted a baby soon. But we've been trying for months with no luck, and I don't want to ruin the trip with the disappointment of a negative test.

Still, I throw a couple in my bag. No harm in knowing.

We grab cocktails with old friends at a dimly lit tapas restaurant on the first night of our trip. I may not be pregnant, I think, but life is still pretty good. On the winding drive to our Airbnb, I feel like I'm going to throw up. I chalk it up to motion sickness. But I can't get it out of my head. I never get carsick. I don't want to get my hopes up, so I try not to think about it as I cuddle beside my husband that night. The following day, I can't escape the thought that it might mean something. So, I grab one of the cheap tests from my luggage and sneak to the bathroom without saying a word to him. Soon, I am sitting on the toilet, hyperventilating.

I am pregnant again.

I peer at the strip on the counter and wonder whether I've conjured up the second line. I desperately want a baby. I mute anyone who shares a birth announcement on social media. When friends say that they are expecting, I struggle to feel excited. But now that I have proof that it's happening to me again, I don't know how to react.

I can't help but marvel at the timing. Days before I should've delivered my first child, I find out I am pregnant. Christmas may not be so bad after all. I walk into the living room, forcing myself to breathe normally, and tell my husband I want a picture of us together. I put my phone in self-timer mode, grab the tripod I've packed so we can take touristy pictures without bothering strangers, and pull the positive pregnancy test out of my pants pocket. Say what you will about influencer culture, but recording special moments on video will always be worth it to me.

He is elated, but my excitement soon dissipates. I cry because I know better than to dream about the future. I was naively optimistic before and have no baby to show for it. My loved ones will be spared an Instagram-worthy reveal this time. It is vital that tragedy not blindside me again.

After I lost the first baby, I felt embarrassed that I had to correct the record after announcing the pregnancy to the world. I remember thinking I would keep my mouth shut if I got pregnant again. In many ways, I process my miscarriage by being ashamed of my decisions. Blaming myself for sharing too early, telling too many people, even grieving too loudly—all ways I cope with the cruel odds I've been dealt.

I leave Asheville sad I won't experience the naivety of my first pregnancy again. Statistics are of no comfort this time around. But I put it out of my mind and start to share the news with family members. I receive constant reassurance that the outcome will be different this time.

After hearing the heartbeat at my first ultrasound appointment, I tell more people. The unease I felt about being too open the first time hangs over me. Still, I have a gut feeling that I won't regret discussing it. I am nauseous nonstop, canceling plans and cutting back on work because I feel sick. Making excuses is getting old. So, I announce my second pregnancy in the first trimester. This time, there is no polished photo shoot—just a picture of me, my husband, our dog, and an ultrasound photo; we look excited and nervous.

Once the world knows, the fear of something happening to my baby is so tangible that I feel like it's choking me. I am so focused on my baby that I never wonder what the worst-case scenario looks like for me.

The pregnancy treats me well, although the first few weeks are tough. My nausea is so severe that I stick barf bags in the glove compartment of my car and try not to gag at the taste when I place Zofran pills under my tongue. I tell myself it is a small price to pay for a baby. In the beginning, I loosely pay attention to a virus I keep seeing mentioned when I flip through news channels. When I am fifteen weeks pregnant, the World Health Organization declares COVID-19 a global pandemic.

Suddenly, my doctor appointments are virtual. Instead of an in-person baby shower, I stand in my parents' front yard as masked friends wave from their cars fifteen feet away. My anatomy scan is at the same high-risk center where I learned about the miscarriage, but I have to attend the appointment alone. These inconveniences are just that—inconveniences. My problems pale in comparison to the suffering millions of other people face. But I can't help but wonder if they foreshadow that nothing will be quite what I expect.

I meet with a doula agency a few weeks into pregnancy. Many of the providers are Black, which is a comfort to me. I've been troubled by things I've heard about Black maternal mortality and my likelihood of dying during childbirth. The cost of their services throws me off; I'm unsure whether I can rationalize the price tag. But my anxiety heightens the closer I get to my due date. I have nightmares that something terrible will happen. Hiring a birth doula doesn't erase the possibility of things going wrong, but it can significantly reduce the risk of complications.[1] I decide to move forward.

A nurse breaks the news at one of my doctor appointments: Because of pandemic concerns, I'm allowed only one visitor during labor. There will be no doula. My husband is the only one I'll have to advocate for me. I trust him, but fear creeps in. We watch videos on birth plans together, taking notes and picturing a positive outcome. The calm woman on the screen tells me to try affirmations. I don't think they'll work, but I memorize a few—what's the downside? I'm not usually superstitious, but I make an exception. I write them down. *I will have an uncomplicated delivery. My recovery will be smooth. The baby will be okay.*

If you're Black and pregnant in the United States, you're three times more likely to die from pregnancy-related causes, and your baby is more likely to be born prematurely. When they're finally here, they have higher mortality rates.[2] Giving birth is one of the most vulnerable things you can do; the rawness of the experience is impossible to escape. You prepare as well as you can—hiring help, researching birthing positions, filling your online shopping cart with postpartum supplies. When people ask how you feel, you smile and say, "I just want a safe delivery." All things within control are accounted for, but what do you do with the parts you can't manage, the unwieldy things left up to fate?

Being rich won't save you. A college degree is lovely, but it isn't enough to protect you. High-income Black patients have the same risk of death during the first year post-childbirth as the poorest White demographic.[3] People much more intelligent than I am have conducted studies that show medical racism is often to blame for the subpar care Black patients receive. Nearly half of White medical trainees believe we have less sensitive nerve endings than our White counterparts.[4] It is breathtakingly unfair.

When tennis star Serena Williams wrote about her harrowing birth experience, I couldn't look away from the computer screen. She fought for necessary treatment after hospital staff dismissed her concerns about blood clots.[5] If one of the most successful Black athletes of our time almost lost her life after giving birth, what does that mean for the rest of us? Can you really be surprised if things don't go according to plan—if instead of the tranquil labor you imagined, you have an experience filled with unforgettable trauma? And that's if you survive. No one can fault the Black woman whose only goal is to make it out alive.

ELEVEN DAYS BEFORE

I feel the urge to go to the bathroom in the middle of the night. This time feels different from the usual pee break. I stand up after I'm done and feel a gush; the floor is suddenly soaked. I know my water has broken. I also know that I'm only eight months pregnant. It is too early, but the baby doesn't seem to care. When I call the after-hours line, the midwife tells me to go to the hospital. "You're having a baby," she says excitedly. I feel like I'm going to pass out.

Labor is boring till it's not. I bounce on a birthing ball between contractions and scroll Instagram, providing my Close Friends list with a play-by-play of what's happening. I am not progressing, and they need to induce, inserting a medication inside me. I am in the most pain I've ever felt in my entire life. But it'll be worth it for my baby. I focus on the lyrics of the song faintly playing from my phone and try to breathe. I feel dizzy anytime I remember that she wouldn't exist without the miscarriage, that I couldn't have both of them. This is not the time to process that, I whisper to myself. Finally—finally!—it is time for the epidural I've requested for hours. At this point, I am delirious from not sleeping and the cramping contractions; I jokingly say I want to kiss the anesthesiologist. The medicine kicks in, and the aching fades. I am ready.

What will she look like? Whose nose will she have? We'll know so soon. I allow myself to daydream as a nurse checks my dilation. I have no reason to be afraid. This is everything I've ever wanted. Soon, it'll be time to push, and I'll lovingly hold my daughter. The fear dissipates. Things are going according to plan.

But then, the monitor that keeps track of her vital signs starts making loud noises. My husband, who can see the screen better than I can, looks alarmed. A nurse assures me that things are okay. The *beep-beep-beep* becomes rhythmic, filling the room with the sound every minute. Still, I am not worried. I trust the professionals who are caring for me. She is mine, and I will have her in a moment. Suddenly, a doctor is in the room. I need a C-section.

"The heart rate is not good." She says it twice. I blink, trying to digest her words. I don't know anything about C-sections other than they are major surgeries, and recovery can be brutal. At this point, it's been thirty hours since my water broke. I want to deliver her my way. I'm so close. The affirmations didn't prepare me for this.

Things happen quickly. I am prepped for surgery. A male physician ambles in to explain that the surgery is emergent, not urgent. He is not in a rush. I do not know the difference, nor do I care. Someone brings scrubs for my husband. Soon, I am in a too-bright room. A nurse places a drape over me. I cannot stop crying. She must be okay. She just has to. The room is silent, except for the muttering of the doctors and nurses. I feel pressure, then hear a loud cry. I could collapse from relief. She is here. She is safe.

And I am in danger.

CHAPTER SIX

I Got Lucky

Her husband reports, "I want her to go back to her old self again."
—My Clinical Documentation Record, page 134

I have twelve hours with the phones that line the wall. They say I can use them between 7 a.m. and 7 p.m., and I stare at the clock until it is time. Access to the outside world thrills me—God speaks to me, revealing things beyond my imagination. I need to call my husband so he can relay it to the news stations outside the hospital. Most of my prophecies arrive at night, so I cannot wait to fill him in every morning when they turn on the phones. I run when it is time because I need to be first. The phones are popular, and I cannot get stuck behind someone rambling about how much they miss home. I have more important things going on. This is how our conversation goes.

Me: *God told me I'm in big trouble.*

Him: *I love you and miss you.*

Me: *People are trying to kill me here.*

Him: *Her umbilical cord stump fell off.*

Me: *You don't believe me.*

Him: *I love you and miss you.*

God has chosen me, and they're trying to kill me because I know the truth. I am both thrilled and terrified. And my husband wants to talk about meaningless things! I'm not sure the baby he keeps mentioning is mine, anyway. God sends me dreams; she might only exist in my mind. I have more important things to consider, even if she exists—if she's even real. The hospital is performing experiments on me without my consent—I'd never say yes to this. I have a gnarly wound on my stomach, proof of the abuse. I ask God to help me forget the pain, but it throbs incessantly. And if that isn't enough, I can't escape the other patients—or are they demons? I am desperate to get out, and my husband can only say he loves me. Useless. My partner, my protector—except now I am entirely alone. He doesn't sound the same, anyway; his voice strained instead of strong. Has he been replaced by an actor pretending to be my husband? I have to ask Jesus.

I later realized he was desperately trying not to cry.

I've never known anything like the exhilaration of receiving a new word from God. My mood changes drastically—the hospital notes call me labile. I am happy that I am a prophet. I am sad because something awful might happen to my daughter, who may or may not exist. I am furious at the doctors who are experimenting on me. The fresh wound right under my stomach is validation. I later realize that it is my C-section incision.

My husband needs to know it all. I've talked to him every day for nine years. He is the first person I call when I find a new favorite tea; no trivial fact is too small. Our text conversations are filled with me describing the minutiae of my day in excruciating detail. Of course I want to tell him everything from the hospital. He looks forward to the phone calls, but for another reason. There is a chance something has changed, and I've returned to normal. But I quickly dash his hopes. He cannot get a word in edgewise.

At first, the calls are all I have—but soon, they are a source of frustration. He wants to talk about the baby's sleep schedule. Meanwhile, I am on the run from assassins. He diplomatically tries to validate my fears without telling me they're true, but it doesn't work. I can sense he doesn't believe me. I hang up on him and pace the halls, wondering why he no longer cares about me. Eventually, the nurses turn off the phones when I try to call home. Later, I think about how afraid we both were. I am worried I am going to die; he worries I will lose myself forever. The road to parenthood broke our hearts, but we've always had each other. Now, we have our daughter, yet we are impossibly alone. I am only thirty miles from him, but we are on different planets.

When left untreated, 4 percent of postpartum psychosis sufferers will kill their infants.

A near-perfect success rate is comforting in every instance except this one. I don't learn what postpartum psychosis is until days after I get home from the hospital. My psychiatrist explains my diagnosis as I try to stay awake during the telehealth appointment, drowsy from all the medication I'm taking. Once I feel better, I begin to research the condition, and my heart races the first time I read that statistic.

I'd heard of postpartum depression, and during pregnancy, I worried about it happening. I didn't want to experience depression with a baby dependent on me. I stayed on an antidepressant with the help of my psychiatrist, though I was wary after my first pregnancy, concerned it might hurt the baby. I dutifully read about the warning signs of depression and made a mental note of the ones that stood out to me based on my mental health history: crying, withdrawing from loved ones, loss of appetite, extreme fatigue, suicidal thoughts. I do not want to experience depression again, but I know I'll survive if I do. I watched YouTube videos, skimmed articles, and scrolled through posts on online forums—but nothing could have prepared me for my reality.

Psychosis is uncharted territory. Detaching from reality is a strange thing. It doesn't matter how educated or grounded you are in everyday life. I wasn't on Earth anymore. I simultaneously thought that my daughter wasn't real and that she was the second coming of God. When you're having a psychotic episode, you're at the mercy of your delusions.

What makes someone likely to develop postpartum psychosis? Those with bipolar disorder face an increased risk—something I didn't think I'd ever need to worry about until I was diagnosed with bipolar during this mental health episode. I didn't care at the time, but it later became something that was hard to digest. My so-called advocacy hadn't prepared me.

A family history of bipolar disorder, experiencing a complicated or traumatic birth, and a previous history of postpartum psychosis can also contribute. Sleep deprivation and hormonal changes may also play a role.[1] Before I became fully psychotic, I marveled at the level of energy I felt. Going to bed felt like a waste of time. Now, I see it for what it was: a glaring warning sign.

During both pregnancies, I wondered what kind of mother I would be. I have a type A personality and struggle to go with the flow, cringing when plans deviate from my expectations. My husband knows better than to surprise me. Because of my anxiety, I knew that I'd be protective of her, terrified of what could go wrong, but I didn't know the extent.

Eight days after giving birth, I abruptly stopped trusting the people around me, people who have kept me safe my whole life. I didn't want them near the baby, and I gritted my teeth whenever I handed her over to someone. When I googled "don't want anyone to hold my baby," parenting forums assured me that it was normal. But something felt off. I wasn't merely annoyed or nervous. I felt panicked. I couldn't say why, but my loved ones shouldn't have been there, including my husband. My memories of that time—of my psychotic self as a whole—aren't linear. It bothered me for a while that I could only neatly remember some things I said or thought. Now, I wonder if my brain was protecting me.

The night things turn from strange to worse will stick with me forever. I wake up in the middle of the night, struck by the realization that my husband isn't reliable. I sneak out of our room and grab a notepad. After scribbling to myself for an hour, I reach a shocking conclusion: He's sleep-deprived. This isn't revolutionary for a new parent, but I've just discovered a thrilling secret. I finally have a reason not to trust him. I grab my daughter from her bassinet and clutch her close, whispering that she is finally okay.

My husband keeps an eye on us from our bedroom doorway as I sit on the couch, as far away from him as I can manage. After that night, he tells me I'm not allowed to be alone with her. She is brought to me, and I stroke her face in wonderment while he carefully watches. I hate him for doing this. But he senses the risk before anyone else. The prophecies start soon after.

Mother–baby inpatient psychiatric units are standard in some parts of the world. Patients in crisis are admitted with their infant children. The concept has spread to parts of the United States, and patients in the units are more likely to quickly recover.[2] But I didn't have the option in Florida, which meant saying goodbye.

On a Saturday afternoon, ten days after having my baby, I panic. My gut screams that I need to go to the hospital. I yell that I am going to kill myself if I stay home, growl at my husband to take me to the emergency room right now. He mobilizes quickly—of course he does—and soon, I am on my way. I run toward our front door, not knowing or caring when I'll return. My mood swings and I happily wave to my mother and the baby as I step outside. An onlooker might think I was heading for a quick walk. The day she was born, it broke my heart to think about leaving her to take a shower. But now, I am too far gone to care. There isn't the tearful goodbye you'd expect of a brand-new mother forced to leave her child. I feel euphoric by the time I climb into the backseat of my father's SUV. I don't grasp the enormity of what is happening or how it'll change my life.

Why was I so eager to be admitted? Everyone around me was adamant that hospitalization would only happen if there was no other choice. I was a new mother recovering from surgery, and it was the height of the pandemic. Leaving home sounded like a nightmare. But that hard-to-place fear that led to me threatening suicide felt like a warning from within, a premonition that things were going to get worse soon. And they did. The hallucinations began moments after my family members walked me to the emergency room. I screamed for help, and someone sedated me within minutes. What would have happened at home? I didn't fully let go of reality until I was somewhere I could receive medical care. Maybe my mind protected me in the midst of its betrayal.

My husband had recorded a video when the nurse brought my daughter to me for the first time after her birth. I am crying, overwhelmed with love for the tiny, perfect human in my arms. You can hear me tearfully whisper, "My baby." The bond I felt from the start is so intense that it almost scared me. So, it's no surprise that people assume they know the answer when they ask the most challenging thing. "I can't imagine spending that much time away from my child," they tell me pityingly. The presumption makes sense, but it's an incorrect one. The separation isn't the most complex part—it's that for much of my time in the hospital, I didn't care.

I can't pinpoint when the delusions started to wear off, but my symptoms slightly improved twelve days after my admission. As I returned to myself, I spent almost all my time thinking about my baby. The phone calls with my husband were less frantic; I didn't interrupt him when he told me about how she was growing. As I fall asleep in my hospital room at night, I chant her name to myself again and again. It is more of a prayer than anything I learned in church. She's real, and she's mine, and one day I'll see her again. I fill a page in one of the notebooks I'm using to keep track of the prophecies I receive, writing her name over and over. I finally have a reason to care.

I had crafted a straightforward maternity plan. I'd take eight weeks away from work, which isn't enough time, but it's all I could afford as a self-employed freelancer. I pictured myself getting lost in new books during late-night feeds, the nursery lamp illuminating the pages. Of course, my days would be spent entertaining visitors as I snuggled my baby. I'd fill my Instagram feed with relatable but curated content, writing captions about how postpartum is challenging but still blissful. Even as I prepared for the possibility of postpartum depression, part of me believed nothing would go wrong. I'd been through enough.

After the psychotic episode, I realized how many people have the experience I assumed would be mine. It's so unfair, beyond comprehension, that some people get to have a baby without extreme suffering—easy pregnancy, ordinary birth story, uneventful postpartum. Outwardly, I'm happy for them. I mean, what else can you be? Deep down, jealousy rages. When someone's story is filled with trauma, I feel better, and I despise myself for it. During these conversations, I hyperfocus on whether I could've prevented my breakdown. If I'd gotten help sooner, would I have suffered so much?

CHAPTER SEVEN

The Doctors Saved My Life

Chief complaint: "I am being held hostage here."
—My Clinical Documentation Record, page 339

The doctor has striking brown eyes and speaks in a gentle tone. I will google him later and would not be surprised to learn he has a dozen five-star patient reviews.

Unfortunately, he is Satan. This revelation comes to me one morning as I sit in the common room of the ward, waiting for God to share more. He seemed perfectly pleasant when I first met him, so it is disappointing that Dr. Ramirez is working against me. God tells me that he has a message for the doctor. I hurriedly write, "I know what you did!" and leave it on the desk in the office where I am evaluated every day.

Because he is Satan, the so-called psychiatrist is also overseeing the hospital's illegal experiments. The doctors at the hospital hold secret meetings to figure out how to bring down people with special powers; at least one other patient on the ward also hears from God, although I'm not sure I believe her proclamations. Also, some nurses are patients in disguise, trying to trick me. They aren't doing this independently; Dr. Ramirez has engineered the whole thing to mess with me.

I don't know who I can trust, so I refuse to take my medication. You would, too, if it might poison you. Although I'm already dead, so how could I be poisoned? Wait. I'm not dead yet. I am in a coma. My family is holding a prayer vigil outside the hospital, and thousands of people have joined. The movement has gone viral, and they are surrounded by news cameras. My network of choice, CNN, has flown in reporters to cover the phenomenon. Before the coma, I was a famous writer. This is why everyone cares that something has happened to me. Every single person in the world is praying for me to get better—even people who aren't Christians. This is a miracle.

But I can't even enjoy the great news because I'm surrounded by people who want to kill me. This isn't a real hospital, anyway. It's hell's waiting room, where you go after you die. God decides whether you'll burn for the rest of eternity, but he has to give you a second chance. My first test is stopping Dr. Ramirez and his staff from murdering us. If I do that, God will welcome me into heaven. I cannot decide whether going to hell or being harmed by the doctors is a bigger problem. Oh well.

Wait. I'm not dead yet. I'm in a coma. How can I be murdered if I'm already dead? Am I dead? Why am I in hell's waiting room if I haven't died? The thought fills me with terror. Will I be the first person sent to hell alive? Dying scares me, but burning for billions of years is especially horrifying. WAIT! There is good news. This is another test from God. I must go to hell and preach the gospel of Jesus. Then, God will save us all. If I thought I was famous before, I haven't seen anything yet. I'll save everyone. Send me to hell, please. I am ready. Ramirez is going to try to stop me, but I'm not going down without a fight.

It's what I've always known. Doctors are evil.

THREE YEARS BEFORE

My fingers tremble as I dial each digit. *8-0-0-2-7-3-8-2-5-5.* The suicide hotline.

The woman's voice is soothing. I guess she has to be.

She asks me what's going on, and I pause. How do I explain that my problems feel small and insurmountable simultaneously? Life is good, at least on paper. I'm spending my days filing stories for a popular digital media site and my weekends exploring our city with my friends. But it is not enough. Depression is here, and this time, it has stayed a while.

My husband is at work. I am so sad. The nice woman tells me I need to seek help tonight. Okay, I think. We will go to the hospital when he gets home and tell them I'm struggling. Maybe they'll give me medicine to help. I take an antidepressant, but I don't think it's working. Do they have counselors on call? I text him that I need the emergency room. He drives home the second he sees my message. Then, we leave.

I am in an intake room, having flashbacks to my hospitalization in college. This time, I won't be spending the night, thankfully. I just need to talk to someone. But once I say I've been thinking about dying, the energy in the room shifts. "You are going to be admitted," they say. I start to cry. I need to go home with my husband, I say in a level voice so the bearded man standing before me knows I'm not deranged. How stupid of me not to realize the hospital would want to keep me. I cry harder, raising my voice as I try to explain how much I want to leave. "You are a liability to the hospital if you leave and something happens to you," the man tells me. I hate him. I cannot calm down. I see a needle. "This might make you tired," drones the man, who is now my enemy. Him and his stupid beard. Soon, I am drifting off to sleep.

The unit is crowded and miserable. My husband comes when visiting hours start and does not leave until they kick him out. I lie in bed despondent. I do not know if I will ever go home. The doctor stops by my room every day for such little time that I never catch his name.

I cry in the common room. A nurse derisively asks me why I'm depressed. "You have people who love you," she tells me. I get the impression from her tone that this isn't true for all patients. I stare at her. Everything in the ward overwhelms me. A blaring television cuts to breaking news. A gunman has killed dozens of people at a music festival in Las Vegas. I plug my ears and hum to myself to block out the noise. Finally, I ask a nurse to turn off the television. I arrive on a Saturday. The days drag on, but Tuesday arrives, and I find out I'm going home. I try to look excited. I do not feel much better than I did when I walked in, but I know better than to say anything out loud.

I tend to respect authority to an annoying degree. When I visit a doctor's office, I am a star patient, hurrying through paperwork like I'll get a medal for filling out my medical history faster than everyone else. I am deferential when I am around people who know more than I do. I've publicly sung the praises of the hospital back home that treated me four years ago. Now, my blind trust in the medical system is gone. Not everyone is on my side.

TWO YEARS BEFORE

She introduces herself with a warm smile. "I'm Dr. Garza," she says. "Nice to meet you, Ayana."

I sit in her dimly lit office, unimpressed. I'm not in the mood for a new psychiatrist on top of everything else I'm dealing with. My husband quit his megachurch job a few months ago, and we are living in my parents' guest bedroom because we need to save money. It feels like I am fourteen again, and not in a carefree way. My mind is not where it should be, and I need a doctor.

One of the only good things about moving home is being closer to Dr. Lewis, the physician who treated me in my early twenties. When I return, she informs me that she specializes in adolescent patients now, and my face falls. I did not expect this to be our last appointment. She scrawls Dr. Garza's name on paper and sends me off. I am in no hurry to meet the woman, who admittedly seems impressive—a quick Google search finds that she completed a fellowship at Harvard. I call and add my name to her patient waitlist.

I'm not holding my breath that I'll find a doctor who I'll like. Dr. Lewis is unusually good, and I won't ever find another version of her. I feel dramatic, but I cannot help but mourn. My experiences since I left her office haven't been pleasant. My last one was awful. He rushed me out of our appointments after the allotted fifteen minutes, regardless of how poorly I was doing. When I found the courage to share that my mood was deteriorating, he responded with little sympathy. Why did he become a doctor in the first place? I suppose the pay must be worth it. The psychiatrist before that was even worse—always late and looking bored when I talked.

I just need someone who accepts my insurance and provides scripts on demand.

Once I start to listen, I can tell Dr. Garza is different. She talks so fast that it's hard for me to keep up, but I want to follow every word. She makes note of my symptoms and suggests a medication change that will help me. Most important to me, she is hilarious. I laugh out loud at her off-color quips. I wish we could bond over drinks even though she is fifteen years older than me, and I'm pretty sure that would break some ethics code.

I leave her office and wait for the elevator, lost in thought. By the time I make it home, I feel hopeful. I can tell Dr. Garza genuinely loves her job. She strikes me as the type to work nights and weekends because she cannot escape her passion. And now she is treating me.

I've been unlucky with doctors in the past. Consider that I was admitted against my will—in my opinion, wrongly so—only a year ago. I lucked out with my first psychiatrist, but the ones I've had since then? Not so much. But I feel a cautious optimism, like I'll finally have someone who cares for the first time in years.

Every corner of hell's waiting room smells like death. I hold my breath as long as I can, but eventually, I am confronted again with the horrific odor. This is the proof I've been looking for. Not only is the hospital running cruel experiments on patients, torturing us for no reason, but the doctors are also killing us. God hasn't prepared me for this.

I ask him for the bravery to investigate further. Suddenly, he tells me to go to the shower room. I open the door, and the stench hits me. I gag, afraid that I am going to throw up.

The smell is awful, but it is far from the worst thing I am experiencing. The shower is filled with dead people piled waist-high. I cautiously get closer, but I cannot hide my terror. This isn't my first encounter with a dead body—I have attended family funerals, politely keeping my distance from the lifeless person in the casket—but it is the only time I have seen rotting flesh. God trusts me with a lot, but this is too much.

As I approach, I concentrate on the faces frozen in terror. To my horror, I realize they are patients. I have wondered where people are disappearing to, and now it is unfortunately clear. God told me that patients leave when it is time to go to hell. He must not have realized the hospital's power to kill them beforehand. I grieve the loss. I start to yell, horrified at what I'm seeing. I knew people were going missing.

The so-called nurses have been asking me if I want to take a shower, and I knew it was a bad, bad, bad idea. I just couldn't place why. Now, I know. If I ever come back to this room, I will die.

But aren't I already dead? Not important, Ayana.

I mourn. I am mad at God. "I never asked to be your prophet," I tell him angrily. "Why did you send me to this disgusting place?"

This is yet another one of Ramirez's cruel tricks. He killed those patients just to make me mad. My anger blinds me. I am ready for

God to give me permission to harm him. He has taken so much. I think of all the psychiatrists I've seen since college. Even the bad ones weren't this wicked.

God smiles. I always feel chills when he smiles at me.

You were born for such a time as this, he reassures. Nothing is impossible.

He always knows best.

I ask God for a message to relay to Satan. He eludes me. Sometimes, he takes a break from talking. I am upset when he goes quiet, but I never let him know. I don't want to seem ungrateful.

Oh, wait. He can read my thoughts.

Damn.

Sorry for cursing, God.

THREE DAYS BEFORE

Dr. Garza is worried.

She has been my psychiatrist for nearly two years, and I adore her as much as I did the day we met. Dr. Garza has been firm with me when I needed it. She rejoices when I share the news of my pregnancy and mourns the miscarriage. Humor remains her forte, and I am still quick to giggle at her jokes. I have seen a range of emotions from her.

But I have not seen this.

I am on the couch surrounded by my family. She sits in her home office on the videoconferencing app we use for appointments.

Everyone is tense. I am having the time of my life.

My psychiatrist listens as my husband explains the concerns. "She's not sleeping," he says, "but she's full of energy."

I interrupt him. "I don't need to sleep anymore," I explain to her. Having a baby has ignited something within me.

She looks at me intensely. Then, it is his turn to talk again. She asks him questions about my mood; my mind wanders as he responds. I am bored, bored, bored. I wish I were talking to my friends, but my husband took my phone away like I was a middle schooler who talked back to a parent. Earlier today, I asked one of my friends to fly to visit the baby today. She has two kids and is expecting another; I do not care that she'll have to drop everything. I need to see her.

Dr. Garza is surprised when my husband shares this tidbit. "You're asking your pregnant best friend to drop everything to come visit with a few hours' notice?" She says it like I'm doing something wrong.

Yes, I say, because "duh" feels rude.

When I look up, concern is written all over her face. I am annoyed. I've never felt better. All my depressive symptoms are gone, gone, gone. We should all be rejoicing, but no one is happy for me. What's that about? She says things like "out of character" and "could be serious." The conversation continues to bore me. I think about taking a lap around the block to get out all the excess energy I am feeling. I've never been a runner, but there's no bad time to start. I fidget, ready to grab my sneakers, then remember I had a C-section less than a week ago. Right. I hear her say *bipolar disorder*. Apparently, my behavior fits the criteria for a manic episode. It barely registers.

I do not understand why I need an appointment with Dr. Garza. Psychiatrists are for when you are sad, and I've never been happier. I am mad, though. Sleep is useless to me, I have realized. I don't need it anymore. All the people who told me sleep deprivation after giving birth would be hard are liars. Why scare a new mom? I make a note to post about this on social media if he ever gives me my phone back. I tune back in just in time to hear my doctor ask my husband to keep her in the loop if things worsen. I am incredulous. Worse? Things have never been better. Has everyone lost it?

The next day, I am no longer incredulous. Life is very, very bad. My baby and I are in danger. My husband and my mother are strangers.

I don't trust anyone inside my house, but I need a favor. I ask my mother to let me borrow her phone, promising I'll only use it to call my father—because my husband took mine, I have no other way out. When she obliges, I frantically dial Dr. Garza's number. Mercifully, she answers. I trip over my words, trying to say them before I'm overcome by emotion. "No one in my life is on my side, and I need help," I rush out as I pace our front porch in my pajamas. I do not know what kind of guidance I need, but I know I can put my faith in her, at least for now.

She asks to talk to my husband. I go inside, give him the phone, and warily stand in the doorway. He is holding my baby—she is no longer *ours*—and it is unbearable for me. He puts Dr. Garza on speakerphone, and I listen. "She didn't sound like this yesterday," she says. "If it gets worse, she may need inpatient treatment." I am stunned. Everyone has betrayed me, including the only doctor I trust. I can't believe her.

I'll die a slow, agonizing death, writhing on the floor until my body gives in if I take the pills. The staff filled them with chemicals that'll kill me. I know this deep down in my heart. But the nurse patiently explains that they'll help me, and I feel an unexpected pull. The day-shift nurses are angels, but the night shift is made up of demons in disguise. It's the middle of the day. I can trust her.

Is it worth risking my life? What does it take to feel better when I'm already dead?

I take the cup. I feel wonder when I look down at my hand. It feels like I'm holding seashells from the beach. One round one that reminds me of butterscotch. A light pink capsule similar to my favorite nail polish color. Tiny blue tablets. Could Satan create something this beautiful?

I believe God, but maybe I misheard him on this one. Besides, I'm exhausted. Death doesn't sound so bad, and dying a martyr means I'll definitely go to heaven. Am I dead? I can never remember. I wash down the handful of pills with apple juice and wait. Nothing happens. I'm not dying.

If God got this wrong, what else is he lying about?

A few days later, I line up at an open door in the ward and wait for my turn to get medication. Earlier today, a doctor told me that I might get out soon. I count the pills before swallowing them. My baby girl is all I can think about. God hasn't talked to me much today. I feel guilty that I haven't thought of him in a while. But I'm so distracted by the thought of a reunion with my daughter that I don't care.

I go to my room to look for a notebook that isn't full and write, "DR. GARZA SAVED MY LIFE!!" in red marker. In smaller letters I add, "Thank you. I hate that it took so long to see it." Under it, an addendum: "This is a REAL psych hospital with real doctors."

For once, my handwriting looks steady. I've forgiven her for betraying me by taking my husband's side and recommending this hospital. They say she'll be my psychiatrist again when I go home. We'll meet weekly until I improve. I'm excited to see her.

At one of our appointments, Dr. Ramirez slowly explains that I've been having delusions, like he's afraid I won't follow his train of thought unless his voice is at 0.5× speed. I still don't like him, but something about what he's telling me makes my stomach ache. The electrifying thrill I get when God tells me to write is the best feeling in the world. I'd give it all just to hear his voice. Just a few days ago, God told me I was the most talented person to ever live. He was so kind to me that day. Reality is blurry. Are my books sacred? I would've bet my life on it.

I can't help but think of my long, complicated history with faith and how it intertwines with my current situation. I spent years praying for a miracle, convinced God would help me because the Bible said to expect it of him. I didn't need to see a doctor because God is both all-powerful and in charge of the universe. He would save me from myself. But he didn't. So I ended up on psychiatric meds—a move that was years overdue—and my skepticism toward the medical establishment dissolved. Suddenly, I trusted the doctors. Maybe even more than I trusted God.

But my faith in the medical system dwindled when I showed up at a hospital for help and ended up being admitted against my will three years ago. When I couldn't find a doctor who valued me as a person, my optimistic views faded. Dr. Garza changed everything by genuinely caring. But she betrayed me when she said I needed to go to the hospital a couple of weeks ago—even though I eventually agreed. Now I've got Dr. Ramirez, who I think might actually be a good man, even though there are still voices telling me to be careful. My convoluted journey could've been avoided if God had answered my prayers when I was a child. I still don't know why he ignored me then but talks so loudly now. My thoughts are everywhere. I don't know what to believe.

I hope God isn't mad at me.

CHAPTER EIGHT

The Pretty Prophet

She is still very disheveled and unkempt.
—My Clinical Documentation Record, page 395

I sit cross-legged in my dark hospital room, begging God for an answer. I need the name of the book I've been writing that feels like it's been brewing my entire life. He says it's not time yet, but I'm consumed by impatience. Could I convince him to tell me?

Suddenly, I feel electric. I can't stay still. Joy overwhelms me. It's always a sign that a word from him is coming. My arms tingle as I raise them, ready to receive whatever he wants to tell me. I grab a notebook and a pencil from under my pillow.

God tells me he wants my help picking a title. This is so exciting that I can't bear to sit down anymore. I walk in small circles around my room.

Stairway to Heaven, he says.

Meh, I respond. Has he forgotten about the Led Zeppelin song?

Okay, he laughs. What about Meeting God?

Too direct, I say. We need intrigue.

I love how honest I can be with him.

Last one, he declares. The Pretty Prophet.

I feel peace. This is it. I write it down in my journal quickly so I won't forget it.

I chose this name, God smiles, because you are beautiful. Soon, everyone will see.

I am gorgeous. He's shown me that.

SIXTEEN YEARS BEFORE

A boy at school—one of the cute ones—asks me about my favorite animal. I do not remember what I told him, but I will never forget his response. "Maybe you should choose an emu instead," he says with a gleam in his eye. "Because they weigh a thousand pounds. Like you." I can tell by the look on his face that he wants to hurt my feelings. A clever comeback escapes me, so I whip around in my seat, returning my attention to our social studies teacher. It is the first time a man makes me feel small, but not the last. The next time my family visits a Publix supermarket, I sneak to the side and weigh myself on one of the giant scales the store is known for. The needle lands on a three-digit number. I am devastated.

I journal through my prepubescent angst, shying away from more serious topics in case anyone finds it. Food becomes a focus. I am offered a slice of cheesecake at a family dinner, I write, but it has seventeen grams of carbs. I write, "SPARE ME!" and underline it twice. When my family prints pictures from a family vacation to Universal Studios Orlando, I can barely look at them. My chubby body is repulsive when viewed unposed from the side. I am mad at everyone for letting me do this to myself. I think I have let myself go, forgetting I am a child. Every Friday after school, I climb into my mother's car and pick out a treat at a dingy convenience store to celebrate making it through another week. The ritual is a favorite. My go-to is a six-pack of Hostess Crunch Donettes Donuts—but that's not allowed anymore. Only skinny people get to eat like that, I tell myself.

THIRTEEN YEARS BEFORE

I sneak into my parents' bathroom, searching for the glass scale by the toilet. I don't know if I'm allowed to weigh myself, and I don't plan on asking. It's much easier to do it when they aren't at home. As I step on, I hold my breath and suck my stomach in like the scale might punish me if I relax. When the number flashes on the tiny screen, I cannot believe it. Let's try again, I think. This time, I strip down naked before weighing myself. The number is the same. Bile rises in my throat.

No wonder I can't get a boyfriend. I storm to my desk, find a black ballpoint pen, and write the digits on my palm, small enough that no one else will notice but large enough to glance at my weight whenever I get hungry. I commit to at-home workouts, repeating the number to myself with each repetition. This is how you win. I will eventually think back to my weight with envy, yearning for the days I was that small.

ELEVEN YEARS BEFORE

We are at a nice restaurant, the kind with multiple dollar signs on Google, on a Sunday afternoon. Our table offers a waterfront view that people ooh and ahh over. I cannot focus on anything other than the plate on the table. I have gained weight—of course I have—and the sandwich in front of me is tempting. I didn't eat breakfast, and I am so, so hungry. I give in to temptation. Regret floods in.

I excuse myself to the ornate restroom, picking the stall farthest from the door, and wait until a chatty group of women enters, their voices echoing through the bathroom and covering up the sound of what I plan to do. I brace myself, then force myself to stick a finger down my throat. Nothing happens. I do it again, reaching deeper this time. I gag. I try again and again and again but can't bring myself to throw up. I exit the bathroom and return to the table with a strained smile. Thankfully, no one asks what took me so long. I can't even do this right.

EIGHT YEARS BEFORE

Grabbing fast food from the student union between classes and milkshakes when I should be asleep are near-sacred rites. College leaves me too busy to worry about what I'm consuming. Having fun is my focus, not my diet. When friends invite me to eat with them, I say yes without hesitation. I feel free. But then I go home one weekend and weigh myself, and suddenly, my attitude toward food is much less casual. An app on my phone gives me a place to log every bite I consume. I contemplate adding chewing gum, even though it's only five calories. Soon, the app is all I think about. It becomes a game. There's a line graph that tracks my weight loss over time. I need it to be as steep as possible.

I research the minimum calories needed to survive.

Months later, I am in a bright clothing store with too-loud electronic music blasting through speakers. I see a pair of pants, but the only size available is smaller than mine. I pick it up anyway and pleasantly ask for a fitting room. I pull them over my legs, then my thighs, then my hips. I button them and take a selfie in the minimalist mirror, so proud of myself I could weep. I do not particularly like how the pants look on me, but they fit. I buy them.

SIX YEARS BEFORE

I look forward to the appointments with my psychiatrist, but I dread the point I step on a scale and watch the nurse write down my weight on a sticky note. I could ask her to hide the number, but it feels silly and attention-grabbing. Usually, I try to tune it out—my relationship with my body is the healthiest it's been in months. This time, I peek. I almost gasp. It's been a long time since I weighed myself—for once, I am doing the smart thing—and I am stunned at how much I've gained. I say all the right things during my appointment with Dr. Lewis. She does not bring up my weight. Still, the number won't leave me. A decade later, I will recall it as easily as my name. When I get home, I pull up a BMI calculator and type in my height and weight. *Obese*, it spits out at me. I am *fat*, I think. For me, it is not a neutral word.

DURING

I am struck by God's kindness. He's been telling me I'm beautiful this whole time, and I finally see it. I will worship him for eternity.

※

Once God reveals the book's name, I am obsessed with The Pretty Prophet.

It's about more than physical beauty, of course. God told me so. If the book is going to replace the Bible, it can't be all about how beautiful I am. Who wants to read that?

But I am beautiful. That's important, too, and I can't leave it out. I haven't believed it my entire life, but God showed me. He calls me lovely. Who could ever talk to him and not want to worship him forever? I don't understand it. How did I make it this far in life without obsessing over him day and night?

Inspiration hits. I have no choice but to stop what I'm doing and hunt for a pen and paper. God keeps me up at night, my mind flooding with new ideas. The Pretty Prophet *will bless billions of people. It'll automatically download onto every phone in the world once I finish writing it, and God will translate it into the reader's native language. News stations will interrupt broadcasts to share the text with their audiences. Parents will teach their children. No one will have to buy the book—this is what makes it more successful than the old Bible. God messed up when he didn't make that one free. Having to pay for the Bible doesn't make sense.*

I stand in my room and examine myself. I look down at my stomach, covered with fresh silver stretch marks from pregnancy. Actually, I'm not sure if that's where they're from. Note to self: Ask God if the baby is real. I think I've checked, but I can't remember his answer. My legs and the cellulite I've always hated. My arms that jiggle if I'm not careful about how I hold them. I have spent so much time contorting my body into a smaller shape. Avoiding mirrors because I don't want to feel disgust. Skipping meals because the thought of nourishing my body is too much to bear.

Not anymore.

God loves it all, and so do I.

FIVE YEARS BEFORE

The dress has champagne lining and a slight train, with floral appliqués adorning the bodice. It is the first one I try on, and I know it is right when I look in the mirror.

Today, it is time to make it perfect. I stand on a stool in the alterations studio, peering at myself in the mirror. I'm in the heaviest garment I've ever worn, but I feel naked. Soon, I'll stand in front of 150 of my closest friends and family members and promise my life to my fiancé. The process has been long—picking the perfect photographer, touring venue after venue, and hiring our wedding planner. The current question is whether I'll think of my "something blue" in time. The dress has never been the most essential part of the process, but it feels like it right now.

I try not to squirm as the seamstress pokes and prods. She alternates between measuring and tugging at the dress. I will look perfect on my wedding day, no matter what it takes.

She looks at me. "It would help if you lost some weight ahead of the wedding. For the dress," she says in a no-nonsense tone.

I thank her, although I feel humiliated. But I'm also grateful to her—appreciative that she confirms something I knew deep down. I am not small enough.

When I get home, I ask Google how to lose weight quickly. I stumble upon a pixelated image on Pinterest that spells it out plainly. NO DESSERTS. NO SUGARY DRINKS. NO REFINED CARBS. NO ALCOHOL. NO ARTIFICIAL SWEETENERS.

I can do this.

I commit to the plan. I tell my fiancé everything, so he knows about this, too. He hates it and tells me so plainly. "You are perfect," he insists. It is a meaningless platitude. No one is perfect, after all.

I allow myself to slip up occasionally, but only occasionally. I imagine my wedding day when I feel tempted to have an iced coffee, extra cream. How do I want to look in the pictures I'll eventually show my grandchildren? At restaurants, I hesitate before ordering. Is the bread really worth it? *I'll have the house salad, please.*

It is Thanksgiving. Our house overflows with the people we love. But my focus is elsewhere. My mother's famous pumpkin pie is on the kitchen table. I love this pie; years ago, I requested this fall dessert for my July birthday instead of a traditional cake. The pie is one of my favorite parts of the holiday. But this year, things are supposed to be different.

I try to bully myself. You'll regret this, the voice in my head says. This isn't going to pay off. The second you finish eating, you will want to throw up. That is how bad you'll feel.

I walk away from the desserts, but I can only think about the pie. I picture how the first bite will taste—smooth pumpkin mixed with sweet cream melting on my tongue. My mind warns me not to do it. For once, I do not listen. Shut up, I say to myself. I get a sliver of pie and savor every second.

The following day, it is time to weigh myself. I cringe. Pie wasn't my only indulgence. Whoever made that Pinterest graphic would have a conniption if they saw my plate: sweet ham, gooey macaroni and cheese, various casseroles, and a vegetable or two to make myself feel better. My progress is probably ruined.

I close my eyes, afraid to open them. To my surprise and delight, my weight is the same. The indulgent dinner didn't affect me at all. I feel a mix of gratitude and discomfort, thankful to my body for not holding onto the food but also wondering whether I need to be doing this at all. Is the restriction even necessary? I wave away the thought.

Three months later, I park my car outside the short, squat building where my final alterations appointment will take place. Our ceremony is only weeks away. I am lighter than the last time I was here.

I slip into the dress, anxiously waiting for the seamstress's response. I need her blessing. In some ways, I did this for her as much as I did it for myself. She appraises me for a while, then nods approvingly. "I'm glad you lost the weight," she tells me.

"Thank you," I beam at her. "Me too."

In no time at all, the day arrives. I wiggle into the most restrictive shapewear I could find. My maid of honor helps me into the elegant dress, and I look at myself in the hotel room's full-length mirror. My hair is perfectly curled, and my makeup is flawless. But the dress disappoints. I could be smaller. I *should* be smaller. Why didn't I buy something less fitted? At least I'm not as big as I was three months ago. In an instant, I am happy.

It's been days since my last shower because God tells me I will die if I go in there. My hair hasn't seen a brush in a long time. Brushing my teeth is no longer a priority. I avoid reflective surfaces—for some reason, it is a scary prospect—but I am in awe of my beauty. When I finally agree to bathe, it seems like the nurses breathe a sigh of relief. It feels like the walls are closing in while I stand under the stream of water, willing it to warm up. I'm not in a hurry to do that again.

God has taught me a lot about myself and my misconceptions about beauty. People on Earth are so focused on the superficial. At home, my bathroom counter is cluttered with products I found wandering the aisles of Sephora after binge-watching YouTube videos from beauty influencers who seemingly lack pores. If I can't control my weight—and trust me, I've tried and tried and tried—at least my face will look good. I contour my nose to minimize the shape and carefully dab concealer on the dark rings under my eyes. If I leave the house without makeup and see someone I know, it embarrasses me. Before becoming a prophet, I would count down to regular manicures and hair appointments. Now that I'm here, I see how futile it is.

I either fight for my life when dealing with Mean God or am in awe of how good he is when Nice God emerges. There's rarely an in-between. I'm so grateful that he's chosen to reveal how extraordinary I am, inside and out. I think back to the time I spent counting calories, cutting out food groups, and committing to trendy diets that I eventually gave up. I was so lost then. God shows me the right way now.

When my husband tells me I am beautiful, he says it out of obligation. When a friend says the same, they're just being nice. When a stranger voices the sentiment, they pity me.

This is how I lived my life before.

The mirror shows me a different picture from the one that other people see. My hair is too short, my nose could be narrower, and my lips are too big—and that's just above the neck. Looking at the rest of my body, I feel disgust as visceral as when you smell something rotten. No one knows this, of course. Outwardly, I am a crusader for the body positivity movement. "One of the upsides of self-love and body positivity is that my fashion sense has improved," I write in one essay. "Beforehand, I was always shopping for the body that I wanted, which meant clothing that was too tight and languished in my closet or baggy clothing that swallowed me whole."

It's an admirable sentiment, but not one that is true. I still obsess over my clothing size, even as I try to help others avoid the behavior. I am a fraud.

I give up on ever feeling better. My therapist knows who I truly am, but barely anyone else is privy. When she gives me advice, I ignore it. I spend a lifetime crusading to shrink my body and then fighting to accept myself. I am tired.

Then psychosis comes along.

Suddenly, I feel attractive without any qualifications. It's low on the totem pole, of course—my priority alternates between convincing God to take me to heaven and fearing a trip to hell, depending on the day—but it is the best I've ever felt. For once, I don't seek outward praise I won't really believe. I finally love myself, even if my internal dialogue is hard to follow.

God tells me I am beautiful, and that's enough for me. After all, I am writing the Bible, and that's about as special as a person can be. Even Jesus had to rely on other people to write his story. God didn't even talk to the disciples like he speaks to me. I know because he tells me. Finally, I have someone whose word I can trust. He couldn't lie to me even if he wanted to. The old Bible tells me so. Although that book will soon be replaced with mine. Maybe God can lie? I need to ask him about it.

Psychosis is a monster. It steals the time I should've spent with my daughter at her most vulnerable age. The condition destroys my sense of self and grasp on reality. When I make it out, I fall into a deep depression—and who can blame me? I thought I'd had my fair share of trauma before the experience, but we are sadly reacquainted. Still, when I lose my mind, I gain something invaluable. I am pretty in a way I never realized. For the first time, my love for myself no longer depends on my dress size.

Talk about a silver lining.

FIVE DAYS AFTER

I pull out the scale after the hospital releases me. Recovering is my ostensible focus, but I can't stop thinking about my body. On the ward, I lost weight—this much I can sense. My shorts are baggy, my face looks hollower, and my double chin is less of a worry. I can't stop wondering how much. I complete the ritual of waiting till early morning, before I eat anything. I am thirsty in the middle of the night, but I avoid drinking even a sip of water, just in case it affects the result. I strip down and pray the scale will be kind to me. I feel a thrill when it tells me I have lost weight, just like I suspected. I don't stop to consider the dark reason the pounds fell off me.

In the hospital, I was convinced that nearly everyone wanted to kill me. Both the pills and the food were filled with poison, so I refused medication and meals, scared of dying. The hunger didn't bother me; I had more important things to do. The delusions led me to the September morning when I was ecstatic about the lost weight. I couldn't spend too much time thinking about how twisted this was. But deep in my soul, I felt it sting.

A week hasn't passed in nearly two decades without me thinking about my body. Sometimes, it is multiple times a day. Even when I resist the temptation to eat too little, I am still preoccupied. Sometimes, I am the biggest person in the room, which makes me wince. I am accustomed to wandering into stores and leaving embarrassed when they say they don't carry plus sizes. I've never been a woman that men gravitate toward, which still bothers me even though I have a loving partner. Even at my happiest, my frame is still disappointing. So, losing the weight is a win. The I-am-so-beautiful self-love framework that psychosis gave me is long gone. I wonder whether the weight will continue to disappear. Maybe the medications I'm taking will kill my appetite, I wonder. There may be a bright side.

Instead, the opposite happens. One of the drugs I'm on is known to cause weight gain—when I google it and read the potential side effects, I dismiss it. That won't happen to me. But my psychiatrist increases the dosage, and suddenly, all I can do is eat and eat and eat. Some nights, I get out of bed to stuff handfuls of cookies into my mouth, barely stopping to chew. During the day, I go back for seconds and thirds, eating until I feel sick. Soon, my favorite outfits are pulling at the seams.

Weighing myself is a dangerous game—I know this. But the drug cocktail I'm on is affecting my body. Everything looks saggier when I look at myself in the mirror before showers. So I dig through the bathroom closet for the scale my husband has begged me for years to get rid of and set it on the cold tile floor. I hold my breath while I wait—old habits die hard—and struggle to exhale once the number flashes back.

Suddenly, it makes sense that I am a clothing size larger than the last time I weighed myself. I feel queasy when I realize I weigh more than I did during my last month of pregnancy. I can't find the words to describe how defeated I am. Briefly, I consider stopping the medication, and I hate myself for it. Will I risk psychosis all for vanity's sake? My desire, at least outwardly, is to get better. But can I recover when I can't stand to look at myself? I am furious. Have I not lost enough?

There's little I won't do for thinness.

If you have the sickness, you know none of it is ever enough. We can watch our bodies shrink, shrug off the compliments, and post the progress photos, but there are always more pounds to be shed. When we meet our ideal weight, the goalposts shift. Suddenly, we realize we can never be small enough. We become accustomed to smiling and shaking our heads when offered food, even as our stomachs growl. Noticing when other people lose or gain weight comes naturally; if you're like me, you hate that your criticism of your own body makes you hyperaware of other people's. Exercise is only worthwhile when it burns a certain number of calories; moving our bodies for the sake of enjoyment doesn't appeal to us. We regret the dessert we ate, as if life isn't too short to deprive ourselves of a cake slice. Compliments are always deflected. We cling to insults like life rafts, holding on to every snide comment ever made about our bodies.

The worst part is the shame. We've been dealing with this forever—for some of us, our formative years are saturated with memories of despising ourselves. The sickness has carried us through childhood, adolescence, and adulthood. We have held its hand on our best and worst days, never letting it stray too far. In some ways, it is a friend, albeit a secret, disgraceful one that no one can know about. The stomach flu is almost worth it for the thrill of losing five pounds in two days. We weigh ourselves again and again and again, delighted when a trip to the toilet causes us to lose one-tenth of a pound. When a psychotic break results in a slimmer body, it is a win. Skinniness is the goal at any cost.

Could we get better? Probably. But do we want to?

CHAPTER NINE

Not Scared

She was observed pacing around the unit screaming, boisterous, and threatening staff about suing the hospital.

—My Clinical Documentation Record, page 405

I sense someone standing behind me. When I turn, I feel dread. He's not supposed to be here. I didn't attend the funeral—acquaintances is a generous way to describe my relationship with his daughter—but I recognize him from the obituary shared on Facebook, his smiling face framed by flowers with "In Loving Memory" spread across the top. He's in hell's waiting room with me—what does that mean? He should be in heaven by now. Was he evil on Earth?

"I know who you are," I yell at Mr. Fields. *He doesn't deserve the honorific, even in my head, but I do not know his first name. I try to be menacing, but the attempt falls flat. He looks back at me, a mixture of confusion and boredom on his face. He does not respond. The silence infuriates me more than any answer.*

When it is dinnertime, I pick the table farthest from him and stare, ignoring the plate in front of me. I use a pencil to hurriedly dash off the latest message God has sent me. Mr. Fields is a test from the enemy. No one should believe this man. I'm the only one brave enough to confront him.

THREE YEARS BEFORE

It is early in the morning on a fall day. I'd tell you about the weather, but I'm not allowed outside.

I sit on my bed in the tidy psychiatric unit at a hospital in Fort Lauderdale, Florida. I am here against my will. It frustrates me that daring to show up and ask for help is punishable, but I can't spend too much time on that. I have to get out of here.

The first time I was admitted to a psych ward, there were barely any patients. I found the experience bearable—even pleasant. This time is different. The unit is filled with people who actually need serious help, unlike me. I can't help but gawk at them. They are unruly. When the nurses give them instructions, they don't listen. Some of them loudly mumble unintelligibly, pacing the halls in circles.

This is far from the first time I've been terrified, but it feels like one of the only legitimate instances. Someone could hurt me at any time. I know people with mental health conditions are more likely to be victims than perpetrators of violent crime—I've recited the statistic more than once—but conventional wisdom is gone. When my husband visits, I almost cry seeing a familiar face.

"I need to go home," I tell him. "I'm not like the other people who are here." Thinking certain types of people belong in a psychiatric ward is deeply twisted, but I don't care. I had some thoughts about dying—big deal!—and now I'm trapped with people who are seriously sick. The fear won't leave.

When I venture into group activities in hopes of going home sooner, I always watch my back. Slowly, I get more comfortable. On my last night on the ward, I sign up for a karaoke group, throwing my head back as I bolt out songs with lyrics that escape me now. I am having fun.

But it's not so enjoyable that I forget the danger. When I walk out of the building, I tell myself that I will never return to a psych ward. I will die first. It's dramatic, sure, but I couldn't be more sincere. Untreated suicidal ideation is hell, but I'll endure it before I ever come back here—not having any say in what I eat, when I sleep, which day I get to go home, or when I can see my family. And that's not even considering that the people I was expected to socialize with were scary to me.

Thankfully, I don't need to worry about it. Things won't ever get to that point again, and if they do, it'll be my secret. No one will know, even those I talk to most. I'd rather die than go back. And I'll try to block out the troubling memories of the other patients. Once I leave the hospital, I will think of them with pity instead of fear. They might have to return one day if they can ever leave in the first place, but I won't. I am fully in control.

We must get out of hell's waiting room. That is today's special revelation. He had me here for a reason, but my mission is over now. I pile up my belongings by the exit and grab the door handle, which is locked. A nurse tells me not to do it again. I ignore her. Again, I pull with all my might. The door won't budge. I am furious. I am being held hostage here, and I need to get out.

Then, God gives me an idea that feels wild, even for him, but I want to be obedient, so I comply. I sneak to the red-and-white alarm and think about what he's asked of me. Everyone will think there's a fire, so they'll have no choice but to unlock the doors. The patients—even the evil ones—will be free to return to Earth, and I will remain God's favorite.

Without a moment of hesitation, I pull it. Strobe lights flash. I am happy because I haven't said no to a mission from him yet. The hospital staff rush toward me. I am confused because the day shift is made up of angels, and I love them. But they don't look particularly holy. They look annoyed.

I flail and scream, furious that they've turned off the alarm and ruined God's plan. They will be punished for this, I remind myself. He doesn't like it when people interfere with his will. The nurses tell me to calm down. I scream louder. They carry me to the seclusion room. It's scary here. My legs thrash around, so they hold me down. "This is not what he wanted," I say. My limbs feel heavy after they inject me with a syringe full of something. At least I tried to listen to him. He'll understand.

A couple days later, he tells me to try again. I am ready. Everything plays out exactly the same—me losing it when it doesn't work, the nurses admonishing me, the chemical restraint when I refuse to chill out. I have a vivid mental picture of everyone being set free, streaming out of the hospital and rejoicing the whole time. Why isn't his plan working? For once, I start to doubt him. Maybe I'll be stuck here forever. I brush off the thought. We'll just have to get more creative.

I am a fearful child.

There are the usual things, of course—roaches, frogs, and snakes terrify me. Once, a giant bug gets into our house, and I simply walk out. But some of my phobias are more unusual.

My mother must avoid the lobster tank at supermarkets because I will have a meltdown if I see them. When we need something from the seafood aisle, I grab her hand and close my eyes as tightly as possible, stopping myself from thinking of their claws and antennas. I have an animal card game with a cartoon drawing of the creature. It is enough to frighten me.

When I am thirteen, my parents and nine-year-old sisters convince me to get on a kids' roller coaster at a local amusement park. They have a blast, squealing as the ride twists and turns. I, on the other hand, am miserable. My scream blends in with all the others, but it is one of terror—I am convinced that I will fall off. Ever the teenager, I pull out my iPod and listen to "Bad Day" by Daniel Powter on repeat after the coaster mercifully stops.

Walking into a public bathroom feels like entering a minefield. I train myself to breathe through my mouth and hold my nose to avoid nasty smells. I research which stalls are the cleanest and find that the first one is least likely to be used. From then on, that is the one I wait for. When I see an overflowing toilet, I think about it for months. In my twenties, I decide to try exposure therapy. One of my first assignments is looking at a toilet smeared with fake poop in the therapy office's quiet bathroom. I cry.

If I am home alone, someone might break in and kill me. I beg my parents to leave only when they must and breathe a sigh of relief when they buy a security alarm. I memorize the code and set it whenever I can. Before using the bathroom, I check behind the shower curtain, convinced that a predator may be waiting for me. I never considered what I'd do if they were.

The nightmares are relentless if I watch anything with suspense, including movies made for children. I plead with my parents to let me sleep in their bed after watching the *Smart House* movie on Disney Channel. A babysitter once puts on *Gremlins*, and I could not rest that night.

What elicits the strongest anxiety is the possibility I may wake up in a suspiciously quiet house and find no trace of my family because they've been raptured up to heaven. I, a dirty sinner, will have to fend for myself, even though I'm not old enough to drive and don't have any money. When I call out for someone in the next room, and they don't immediately respond, I have to stop myself from frantically yelling. I behave as well as possible to make sure God won't leave me stranded. (Thanks, *Left Behind* movies.)

Some of these anxieties fade as I age, but many get worse. I still can't handle bugs and shudder when someone at my table orders a lobster tail. Public toilets no longer petrify me, but I wait unless I have no other option, tightly crossing my legs to hold it in on the drive home. On road trips, when there's no choice other than seedy gas stations, I take deep breaths before exiting the car. And of course, I always have hand sanitizer at the ready; simply scrubbing my hands raw in hot water isn't enough.

Still, my biggest fears revolve around how people perceive me. I am a stickler for adhering to the rules. At school, I am the teacher's pet, happy to rat out fellow students who misbehave, and it's a title I wear with pride. I have my first alcoholic drink on my twenty-first birthday. It doesn't occur to me to indulge earlier and break the law. When I am pulled over on the way home from a college internship for driving above the speed limit, I cry so much that the stern cop lets me go out of pity.

This is the course of my life, and I'm not unhappy about it. My apprehension keeps me safe from any consequences that come with living wildly. Sure, life may be more interesting if I was more spontaneous—the kind of person who snuck out of the house in high school or peered at a classmate's Scantron sheet before bubbling in their own—but I'll trade exciting stories for the security that comes with conforming.

Psychosis changes everything. I'm no longer nervous; it's like I've never known panic. I've been set free.

Hell's waiting room is my home now. I'm not sure if I'm sad about this. I miss my family. I think? My intuition tells me they may hurt the baby, which I can't even think about. If anyone harms her, God will murder them. She is Jesus, after all. Nice God is hard to read, but he is always generous. He sends angels to the waiting room to help me conquer the confusion Satan is sending my way. But I also have to look out for lurking demons. Everyone is good or evil, with no exceptions or gray areas. The day-shift nurses are a gift from heaven, but the night shift wants me dead. Nurses don't always stay in their assigned category, and someone who seems honest can quickly become the enemy. It's complicated.

An angel becomes a demon when they don't listen to God or believe his prophet (that's me!). Regrettably, God never gives me a heads-up when someone turns on me—this is one of his tests. I have no choice but to be wary of people. Anyone can flip in an instant. I rejoice when new patients walk into our space between heaven and hell. They usually don't look happy, which I understand. They're probably reeling from the trauma of dying, especially if they thought they'd wake up in heaven. Anyone would be nervous to enter this combat zone. I need them on my side, though. Building God's army is the only way to get out of here. I have to be brave.

Cameron is my best friend. Or is it Casey? I can't remember her name, but that's okay. God sent her just for me. She's an angel, although she's a little rough around the edges.

Cameron has short black dreads and a gravelly voice. We would not have discovered each other on Earth, but she is perfect for the conundrum I've found myself in. She listens when I get a new prophecy and need someone to share it with. I explain which patients are actually nurses in disguise, and she accepts it, never questioning what God is telling me. Everyone I'm supposed to listen to—the doctors, my husband, my parents—they all tell me I'm not hearing from him. I love her. She is my best, best, best friend. We're going to get out of here together with heaven's help. WAIT. I feel a new word coming on.

Did God send her, or was it the devil? Can I trust her? I need to know now.

A horrible thought occurs to me.

Is she, too, a test?

FOUR MONTHS AFTER

I can't forget my behavior and the way I treated the other patients. At one point, Cameron yelled at me that I should be grateful I had family members who still took my calls. I retaliated by accusing her of assaulting me. When the hospital asked if I wanted to file a report, I told them I just wanted to go home. I still feel disconcerted remembering it, like I'm reliving the moment.

I struggle to place the emotions I'm feeling. It takes me a second to fully realize the discomfort. I've become the patient I feared three years ago when I was involuntarily admitted to the hospital for suicidal ideation. Behaving erratically, yelling at people, talking to myself—I wouldn't blame anyone who decided to keep their distance from me. Past Ayana would've felt bad for Psychotic Ayana. She would've wondered whether I was well enough to feel embarrassed. I think about the other patients on the ward during my psychosis stay and what they must've thought of me. Surely, some of them felt the same unease I did when hospitalized for suicidality around seemingly unstable patients.

When other kids called me a tattletale when I was young, I couldn't feel insulted. They weren't wrong. I kept my eyes peeled for troublemakers, not because I liked seeing my peers disciplined, but because I couldn't stand for things to be out of order. I landed in the principal's office during my junior year of high school for arriving one minute past the tardy bell, and I wept when they told me they might call my parents. When fistfights broke out on the main lawn, I'd speed-walk the other direction as classmates pushed forward to get a better look. My contentedness is predicated on never being too loud, disobedient, or belligerent. Some of this comes from me being a Black woman in America, constantly aware that I may be perceived as aggressive and scared of what may happen if I'm hostile. But part of it is just my goody-two-shoes personality. I'm docile until I'm not.

When I pulled the fire alarm, screamed at other patients, and accused people of being demons, I felt alive. Finally, I thought, I have been delivered from the anxiety that's plagued me for my entire life. I would've happily tackled an intruder or killed one hundred bugs while in psychosis. For once, I didn't have to overanalyze every possible consequence before deciding. I was free to do whatever I wanted. Who cares if I got in trouble? I'm God's favorite, and that's more than most people have. My bravado empowered me, even if it scared other people.

I wish I could say sorry to the medical team who helped me, though I'm sure they've seen worse. I am humiliated by my behavior. It doesn't matter that I wasn't in control of myself—if anything, that bothers me more. The voices were in charge, and I didn't dare say no. They could've told me to do anything, and I would've tried it. I once taunted another patient by saying that she wasn't actually hearing from God; he'd told me to warn her, so I had to. When she lunged at me, I felt nothing. If she'd gotten close enough, I would've happily fought back.

Psychotic Ayana is bold and doesn't care what you think of her. She won't let discomfort get in the way of loudly sharing the truth. She is brash and cruel. Psychotic Ayana loudly drops expletives without caring what anyone says, ignoring the fact that she never curses in public. She isn't scared of anything.

That woman is a lot of things, but she isn't me. Not anymore.

I've always hated that I'm so easily frightened. It's embarrassing to hold all your friends' purses and wait behind while they run around a theme park, jumping from roller coaster to roller coaster. Me crying at fake poop is so humiliating that I considered omitting it from this book. And, of course, there's the lifelong panic. Did you know the Bible tells readers to be unafraid hundreds of times? I can quote the verses easily. Me being a scaredy cat isn't just annoying. It's disobedient, and God expects more. I don't think like this anymore, but some remnants still cling to me. I looked longingly at people like my husband, who once offered a "not really" when I asked if he had any fears. What the hell was wrong with me?

Psychosis did what God didn't—or couldn't. The thrill I felt when fearfulness faded away made me feel like I was on drugs, capable of absolutely anything. Cleanliness wasn't constant in the hospital bathrooms, which would've nearly ruined me before, but during the episode, I didn't care. God told me I was flushing out demons anytime I used the bathroom, so I dutifully awaited the urge to go. I didn't hold my breath or avert my eyes. It felt so nice to move through the world like that. Not scared.

The word *brave* is inked on my left shoulder. I was twenty-one when I got the tattoo. At the time, it was a declaration—an act of hope, maybe. But in the years after, I wondered whether it was overcompensation. Someone who's actually courageous doesn't need a permanent reminder of the fact, right? Eventually, bravery found me, and I could finally live without anxiety. What a gift.

It only took me severing my grasp on reality.

FIVE MONTHS AFTER

I stand in our open-plan kitchen and wash our dishes from the day, taking special care with the baby bottles. My husband sweeps the floor behind me with the cheap broom we need to replace. We engage in mundane conversation about our day, the kind of surface-level talk that bored me till the episode deprived me of my ability to have a normal conversation. Now, I don't take it for granted. Suddenly, out of the corner of my eye, I see a large shadow. I jump. The fears of my childhood come rushing back. What if someone is in the house? Oh my god. I spin toward him, my hands shaking.

"Did you see that?" I ask urgently.

"See what?" he responds.

"The shadow in the hallway over there," I say.

Why would someone break into our house? What could they want? I think of the podcasts I listen to on long drives that describe assaults and murders in brutal detail. You should always be prepared for the worst, they tell me. Did my husband lock the door after he got home from work? If he did, how would someone get in? He interrupts my train of thought.

"I didn't notice anything," he tells me.

Before I lost my mind, this exchange wouldn't be worth remembering. A weird one-off, I would think, before turning my attention back to the soapy sink. I'd chide myself for having such an active imagination. This will make for a funny story to tell our friends one day: *Ayana convinced herself she'd have to fight off an intruder!* I'll leave out the parts about my racing heart and genuine terror. But things aren't like they used to be. Lately, I have been afraid of everything. I cannot shake the thought that someone else is in the house, and my baby is in her crib by herself, as vulnerable as can be. I try my best to stop panicking. It doesn't work.

My husband has grabbed the mop, unaware that we might die at any moment. I keep my voice level low when I ask him to check the whole house to make sure no one is there. I stand in the living room and wait impatiently. After a quick sweep of all three bedrooms and two bathrooms, he confirms our sleeping daughter is the only other person here. This should be a relief. I will not die today. And I should probably stop listening to those podcasts.

My fear immediately shifts. If nothing is there, does that mean my brain invented it? My mind works this way these days. When you lose trust in your ability to perceive the world, you second-guess everything. In psychosis, I couldn't tell truth from fiction. I don't dream of saying this aloud because voicing it may make it real, but I can't stop thinking. What if the psychosis wasn't an isolated event? There's a chance my mind is gone again, even though I feel like I'm doing better.

Instantly, the walls of the kitchen start to close in on me. It is happening, I want to scream. It is happening again. Call Dr. Garza. Tell my parents. My baby's wispy hair is reminiscent of her father's. She never stops smiling and laughs when we play music. My love for her is so present that it hurts. I can't lose her again. I collapse onto the ground, crying so hard I can barely breathe. Soon, his arms are around me. The comforting words mean nothing. The hallucinations are back, and I have no way to stop them.

It isn't a fluke that I saw someone. There's no way it could be. It felt so real that I would've bet my life on it. So what does it mean if nothing was ever there?

How foolish of me to think I could make it out of psychosis unscathed. Moments from the hospital when I wore defiance like a badge of honor flash before me. I would laugh if I weren't busy freaking out. I don't know where Fearless Ayana went, but she's long gone.

CHAPTER TEN

A Terrible Hangover

Ayana stated, "I will kill you all. You'll see."
—My Clinical Documentation Record, page 189

THREE YEARS BEFORE

String lights twinkle in the air. It is a muggy Florida summer night—the kind that makes your clothes stick to your back the second you step outside. My friend is having a party, and I am mingling and trying to ignore the stifling weather. The alcohol is flowing. I have a glass of wine; when I finish it, I say yes to a second. I search for food. My head is starting to feel light, and I don't want to get drunk. To my dismay, there's barely anything to eat. I shrug and head back to the party. What can you do?

I have a cup of water before saying yes to a cocktail when it's offered. This isn't my norm. Usually, even being tipsy is too much for me. I don't like sacrificing my composure, especially if I don't have to. Enjoying the occasional drink is fine, but I'm not the person who downs them when I'm out. For some reason, tonight is different.

I'm making conversation—and doing a great job, I might add—when I stop myself in the middle of a sentence. My eyelids are heavy, and my brain feels fuzzier than a dandelion. "Excuse me," I say graciously. "I think I've had too much to drink." I find a chair and sit down. Thankfully, my husband drove us here, and he's not in the same predicament. Once I steady myself, I go back to making my rounds, ignoring that I'm a bit wobbly. When it is time to go, I offer my goodbyes and head to the car. I tell my husband I had a lot of fun.

Then, the next morning hits.

I wipe the sleep from my eyes, and I groan. My head is pounding, and I feel like I might throw up. I am exhausted even though I'm waking up way later than usual. I don't think I've ever felt worse. Getting out of bed feels like a herculean task, but I haven't been this thirsty my whole life. My husband is already at work; mercifully, I have the day off. I crawl to the bathroom in search of Advil. Last night was a mistake, to say the least.

I stay in my pajamas all day, and soon, the sun sets. Incredibly, my head still hurts. I wonder whether I'm going to feel like this forever. (Me? Dramatic? Never.) I have dinner plans I don't want to cancel, so I force myself to get ready. The headache hasn't left when I get to the restaurant, nearly twenty-four hours after the party started.

The physical symptoms, as unpleasant as they are, don't bother me as much as they could. I'm thinking about something much worse: What if I said the wrong thing? I try to replay every conversation and remember exactly how they happened, but the night is blurred in my memory. Did I talk too much? Laugh too loud? I could've told a long story and missed cues that other people were getting bored. The possibilities for embarrassment are endless.

I become fixated. First, I ask my husband whether he noticed me doing anything unusual. He assures me he did not, but that's not much comfort. We were separated for most of the night, socializing with different groups of people, so I could've misstepped without him there. I sit in the loud restaurant and try to keep up with my friends' conversations, but my mind is elsewhere. I can't believe I let myself lose control in public. Why didn't I switch to soda? I know I'm a lightweight. Is this a case of me sabotaging myself? If so, why? The questions keep turning inside my brain.

When I get home to our apartment and flop on the couch, I consider asking another friend who was there whether I acted awkwardly, but I don't know whether I should bring it up. If she wasn't paying close attention to me and I asked her to scrutinize every word she heard me say, I could make her overthink my behavior, which is exactly what I want to avoid. I decide against it.

I can't stop dwelling on it, though. I tactfully decline when I'm offered a drink at the next party. I'm still struggling with how I may have behaved that night. It feels silly to shame myself over something that may not have happened, but I cannot stop.

Eventually, the moment fades to a distant memory. I try to treat it as a funny anecdote. *So this one time, we were at a party, and I accidentally had way too much to drink. . . .* When you tell a story the right way, people will laugh, especially if you're the butt of your own joke. I am reminded of two things I've long known. I hate to relinquish control, and I don't forgive myself easily. I don't know whether I did anything wrong, but that doesn't matter. Keeping my guard up is easy, and not just around alcohol. I'm less likely to humiliate myself if I'm hyperaware in social situations. I figured it out a long time ago. Maybe you've been there, too.

But are we ever really in control? We can analyze every word we say and obsess over other people's approval and take measure after measure to prevent ourselves from creating awkward situations. We can beat ourselves up when we inevitably do the wrong thing, even if the punishment doesn't fit the crime. And, of course, we can spend months—or years, even—convinced that we're the worst people alive over a minor slight. Keeping a mental record of every time we've messed up since childhood is always an option. The goal is simple: bully ourselves into never offending anyone, never expressing an opinion that's too controversial, and never being annoying. And we can get really, really good at it. We might feel like we're in charge. It's exhausting to live our lives this way, of course. But isn't it better than the alternative? Until things go wrong, and we're no longer in the driver's seat. Maybe we have one too many drinks or get too comfortable in a conversation and let ourselves slip. For me, it's losing my mind and grasping to find it again.

When shame and I meet again three years after the party, it's worse than ever.

I stare at my sleeping baby in her bassinet, overwhelmed with awe. I can't believe I made her. She is so beautiful. It's only been a couple of days since I gave birth, but I feel like I've known her my entire life. I pull out my phone and snap pictures of her from every angle. She's wearing a onesie I picked out right after my doctor told me I was having a girl. I'm biased, but she is an objectively adorable baby. And she's so tiny—only five pounds—and looks like she'll break if I pick her up too quickly. I am terrified something might happen to her. Do all parents feel this way about their kids? I set a mental reminder to text one of my mom friends to ask.

I swipe through the photos on my camera roll, deleting a few that came out too dark. Now, there's the question of who to send them to. I dash off a text to my parents and a few close friends, captioning the pictures with "CAN YOU EVEN HANDLE HER?!" Who could blame me for being excited? I staged this photo shoot to share the photos only with loved ones, but now, that doesn't seem like enough. Everyone deserves to see this beautiful baby.

I scroll through my contact list. Names start to jump out at me. A friend from college whom I haven't talked to in years? Check. My psychiatrist at the for-emergencies-only cell phone number she gave me at a recent appointment? Check. My former boss, with whom I am on good, but still professional, terms? Perfect.

Within minutes, I've fired off all the text messages. People respond nearly immediately with variations of "So cute!" I am thrilled. More people should know how precious she is, and now they do.

Isn't it normal to be happy?

Years ago, I'm in a long Starbucks line, standing behind a woman wearing a shirt I love. I compliment her, and we start to chat. By the time it's her turn to order, we are Facebook friends. Nine years later, we still double-tap each other's posts.

My husband and I are staying at a comfortable hotel on the beach for my birthday. Much to his displeasure as a fierce introvert, I love small talk. I am feeling particularly friendly that day. In the time it takes the elevator to reach the ground floor from our room, I make a friend.

I love networking events, the kind with scalding coffee in large dispensers and almost-stale pastries, and I prefer to go alone. Walking into a room where I don't know anyone and scanning the space to figure out who to approach is like a puzzle. I know I'm unbearable, but meeting new people excites me. It's one of the reasons I went to journalism school.

This hasn't always been the case. In childhood, I hid. A book was a better companion than most of my classmates, anyway. I struggled to make eye contact and mumbled answers when I was called on in class. But, tired of fading into the background, I slowly pivoted to extroversion as I got older. I haven't looked back. If Ayana Lage is anything, she is fun.

Outgoingness may imply that I'm laid-back, but it's far from the truth. I obsess over saying the right thing. My conversations aren't as organic as they may seem. No one knows it, but I play a part like an actor in a movie. I carefully read the other person's body language, ask engaging follow-up questions, and crack jokes without seeming like I'm trying too hard. Every interaction is like a job interview, except I'm trying to win friendship instead of an offer letter. My success rate isn't 100 percent, but it's good enough that it's worth playing the game.

Sometimes, it's tiring, but I don't mind. I'm more likely to make mistakes when I'm not overanalyzing everything I do and say. Staying vigilant helps me guarantee that people will want to be my friend, too. I don't always get it right, but I'm socially adept. I struggle to fill occasional awkward silences, and I don't always have the perfect response, but I can pick up on cues. I am confident. Well, kind of. I seem confident to everyone else, and that's what matters.

It's one more thing psychosis takes from me.

I can't put my phone down. Not that I want to.

It feels like I'm talking to everyone I've ever met. Honestly, that's not too far off—every time I think of someone else who might care about my daughter, I text them updates. I've run through my close social network and have moved on to acquaintances. The responses are all polite, which gives me motivation to continue. I call a friend on FaceTime to loudly complain about my husband. My Instagram Close Friends list balloons as I add everyone that comes to mind. I'm always social, but this is another level.

I'm not feeling chummy with everyone, though. The messages I receive from online strangers congratulating me on my daughter's birth are suffocating me. I try to turn off Instagram Story replies but can't figure out how. The tutorials online are too long, and I lose focus. This is frustrating. I excitedly remember that I know someone who works at Instagram. We have talked only a couple of times, but I need help. I immediately email her, and she replies quickly with a simple explanation. I am grateful.

It hits me that tens of thousands of people follow me, and someone in that number could want to harm me. In between blasting out texts, I refresh my email, ignoring the out-of-office autoresponder in place for the next eight weeks. How silly of me to think I'd be able to stay away. A new message pops up from an unfamiliar name. They say they understand why I shut down Instagram replies but wish they could still respond to my posts. This enrages me. My boundaries have been violated. I open the Instagram app and pen a tirade warning people to stay away. If they don't, I confidently write, I'll have my mother reply on my behalf. In my mind, this is the ultimate threat. I do not run my plan by her.

What would make me feel better? What if I deleted all my social media profiles? Went completely off the grid? I stop to consider it, but it feels like an ambitious plan. I shill all sorts of things on Instagram—flavored chips, robot vacuums, my favorite diet soda—and the checks I receive pay my bills. Getting away from the app entices me, but I don't think it's realistic. What else could help me, then? I don't realize I've asked the question aloud until my husband softly suggests I put my phone down for a few minutes. I ignore him.

I return to my phone, open the app again, and scroll. I'm struck by how beautiful all the people I follow are—acquaintances, friends, family, strangers. Soon, my fingers tap away as I comment on nearly every post I see. Eventually, my hand gets tired, and I let go of my phone for a second. It doesn't last long. I am talking on the phone again. To whom? About what? Does it matter? My baby is whimpering in her bassinet, but I'm busy. I ask my husband to check her diaper without looking away from the screen in front of me. My love for her is all-consuming. But I have other things on my mind.

For twenty-one blissful days, my lifelong struggle with anxiety is over. I don't care what anyone thinks, even those whose opinions once meant the world. What strangers say is no longer any of my business. I can't believe I wasted so much time worrying about how others might perceive me. I think about all the little moments that have hurt my feelings over the years: a friend unfollowing me online, no invitation to someone's birthday party, an offhand comment that sticks with me for years. Those anxieties are gone. I wonder why I ever cared. My behavior might be strange, but I just had an emergency C-section after going into labor a month early. And, of course, there's the hormones and sleep deprivation that postpartum brings. Who wouldn't feel a little odd?

How quickly things change. One day, I share a rambling message to my Instagram feed and sign my husband's name. He deletes it thirty minutes later, but thousands have already seen it. (For years, it will keep me up at night.) Then, he asks for my phone. He yanks it from my hand when I don't offer it willingly. He comes up with a new passcode. He changes the password on his phone, too—he knows me well enough to know I'll attempt to use his if I can't have my own.

When religious delusions take over, and the voice of God becomes as familiar as my own, embarrassment is the last thing on my mind. I am at risk, although I won't realize it for some time. But before then, I live without constraints, unaffected by social norms and other people's thoughts. The manic episode is the first time I feel truly free in my whole life. Conversations no longer feel like minefields where I'll blow up if I say something wrong. I don't think about politeness anymore. I've been nice for too long. I'm not careful anymore, which is electrifying beyond measure. It feels like I'm floating, no longer weighed down by my perceived gaffes. No more keeping track of every word I say. For once, I am liberated.

Of course, there is a trade-off. When I stop considering how my actions might affect anyone else, I make decisions I regret. While in the hospital, I scribble "STOP TRUSTING RANDOM PEOPLE" in a journal in slanted, rushed handwriting. This is the opposite of how I usually live my life, where someone's thought of me means everything, even if I don't know them well. I am now unstoppable. There's nothing anyone can say or do that will affect me.

Later, as I read the medical records, I try to comfort myself. At least I'll never see the people from the hospital again. How I acted while psychosis was on the horizon haunts me. The paranoia. The meanness. The overfriendliness with people I barely know. For someone who prides herself on reading the room, it's almost too much to bear. And that's not even the worst of it.

I open my phone to a text from my father that sets me off. I complain to my husband, but he says the message is harmless, infuriating me even more. I know what I need to do. My family will never see my daughter again. I'm cutting them out of my life. He looks alarmed as I relay all this to him. He cautiously tells me I may be overreacting because of a misunderstanding. I cannot understand why he is on their side.

My parents are dead to me. Should I mourn the loss?

I send ten texts in a row telling them this is our last conversation. It doesn't matter that they have been a steady support since I gave birth, coming over to clean our house and hang WELCOME BABY! *signs and* balloons. That my mother dropped all her responsibilities to cook us lunch today. None of it matters. I'm done.

I screenshot the conversation and forward the picture to a dozen people, seeking validation that I've done the right thing. Instead, everyone seems to have the same reaction as my husband. This is what betrayal feels like, I tell myself. I've lost my family, and now my friends are gone, too. I have one friend I can count on, though. We've known each other for years and never disagreed on much. I stare at my phone, waiting for her response. Finally, it comes. The text reply says exactly what everyone else has told me—that cutting ties with my family over a misinterpreted message is a step too far.

I've lost her, too.

I tap the letters out slowly, making sure I don't have any typos. I don't want anything to get in the way of what I need to say. I press the send button. "MIND YOUR F*****G BUSINESS," the text reads.

I throw my phone across the couch and sigh. I've never talked to anyone like this, but it feels . . . good?

I later find out that she quickly reached out to my mother after seeing my response. "Something is wrong with Ayana," she said.

SIXTEEN MONTHS AFTER

The Zoom window takes up my entire monitor. As I wait for the call to start, I try to ignore my escalating nerves. I am wearing one of my favorite sweaters, concealer, and blush, and my hair is pulled into a bun. If you saw me, you might think I was on my way to a first date.

Meeting your therapist for the first time is more important than what any man might think. Ideally, they'll be impressed. "Ayana is so well-adjusted," they'll muse. "Why does she even need therapy in the first place?" If only.

I cold-called the therapy office, asking if any practitioners were available. The cheery receptionist recommended Dr. Jones. "She's great," she said. "And she takes insurance." Her voice dropped like she was telling me a secret. I'm sold. My co-pay is only thirty-five dollars.

She is my sixth therapist in eight years. I know it sounds like a commitment issue, but I struggle to find a provider I can connect with who won't break the bank. Dr. Jones, a Black woman with cropped hair and a warm smile, is a trained psychologist. She introduces herself and asks me to share more about my life.

The question is standard for an introductory session, but I rush through my answer. She doesn't need to know every trauma I've experienced. I only need her to help me overcome everything I said when my brain fell to pieces. I tell her this, and she nods. "What happened?" she asks. I start to cry.

Everything comes pouring out. I tell the therapist about the awful words I flung at my loved ones while they told me how much they cared about me. I cringe when I open up about how I bombarded a friend I'd met weeks prior with text messages detailing my every thought. My phone screen was filled with blue bubble after blue bubble, not caring if I received a response. And I shudder to remember how I asked everyone around me for money—family members, friends, complete strangers on Instagram. The worst part isn't even that I sought it, but that people opened their wallets to give me help I didn't deserve. I think about these things daily, I tell her. Sometimes, multiple times a day. I can't let it go.

She takes a beat before responding, and what she says changes everything.

"You did not embarrass yourself as much as you think you did."

I feel myself freeze, wondering whether it's true. I'm not sure I'm convinced, but I want to trust her. I jot it down so I can reference it later. I'm afraid I'll block out her words otherwise.

I wake up in the middle of the night. I would give anything to know the time, but they don't let me have my phone in the ward, and I don't feel like going to the common room. A new revelation has arrived, and it horrifies me—I am overwhelmed by the stab in the back.

My husband is cheating on me.

This is my biggest fear. He knows this. How could he?

Back on earth, I would've searched for corroboration. Gone through his phone looking for damning messages or grilled him to determine whether he was lying. But now, I don't need any proof. God told me in a dream, so I know it's true. That's the one good thing about being in hell's waiting room, I guess. I have a reliable source.

I dread confronting him. He doesn't lie to me. The only time I remember him fibbing was when he was planning our engagement and wanted it to be a surprise. But if he found someone else, would he really want me to know? Sometimes, I get mad at God for telling me things I wouldn't find out otherwise.

It feels like forever before the phones eventually turn on. I call him at 7 a.m. sharp, eager for his answer so I can figure out whether I want to end it with him. When he answers the phone, I spit my words out with vitriol. I barely allow him to respond before telling him I need to hang up. He sounds weary.

I return to my room and find a notebook. "I'm considering divorce because all we have in common is our love," I write. "It's enough . . . so why divorce him?" I reread the sentences, satisfied they make sense.

I don't know if I'll stay.

Perhaps the friend who Venmoed me twenty dollars when I asked still thinks about it years later, annoyed about the request. My parents could resent me for kicking them out of my life for a day, even though they've told me it is fine more times than I can count. My husband, the best man I know, might still take offense at my agitated declaration that he was cheating on me. My meanness may have turned people off permanently.

Yes, this could all be true. Or maybe I'm being defeatist, and people give me more kindness than I allow myself. The acquaintances I bombarded with pictures of my daughter—they probably understand that I was excited to show her off. Those who sent money looked out for me in a way I didn't think I needed, but maybe I did. They didn't respond because they pitied me but because they saw a tangible way to help a new mother struggling. Sometimes, my therapist tells me, helping someone does as much for the giver as it does for the recipient. So, a person who reaches out may lend a hand because it makes them feel better, too.

The strangers who responded sympathetically to my erratic social media posts were probably genuinely concerned. Sure, at least a few of them may have rolled their eyes at my over-the-top behavior, but most showed remarkable care toward me. I've spent my life assuming that any error will make everyone shut me out, but psychosis showed me the opposite. Viewing myself through an unsympathetic lens, where every blunder is cause for self-castigation, has warped how I see my life. I can beat myself up for decisions I can't go back and change. It's how I've lived for three decades, and it feels like it's worked so far. But maybe I'm selling everyone else short by assuming they think the worst of me. Rather than letting the worst-case scenario consume me, I could just . . . live.

I agonized over whether to say sorry to the people in my life I'd insulted. Text messages and phone calls echoed in my head. No one was exempt—I was astonishingly rude to most of the people around me, including my elderly grandmother. I was ill, but did that lessen the impact of the things I'd said? My loved ones deserved apologies, but I couldn't find the words. A big part of me hoped they'd somehow memory-hole the whole month and forget our conversations. Or maybe they'd put their hurt feelings on the back burner because my mental health was a much more present issue. It may have been cowardly, but I didn't say sorry for most of the things I did. Months after the hospitalization, I found the courage to apologize to my husband for the peculiar Instagram post I'd shared in his name. He assured me he didn't care what strangers thought of him. I wish I could say the same.

I want to think people are too busy thinking about their own mistakes to spend time worrying about mine. It sounds too good to be true, but I don't devote significant energy to other people's faux pas. I can beat myself up and force memories to loop in my head, but for what? It doesn't serve any purpose other than forcing suffering on myself. I've long thought this is the best way to live, but I don't know if I can do it anymore.

Is it really what I deserve?

CHAPTER ELEVEN

Sitting in Silence

She is religiously preoccupied. Always mentioning Jesus.
—My Clinical Documentation Record, page 228

THREE MONTHS BEFORE

He can supposedly stop terrible things from happening—miscarriages, cancer, death, pandemics—and just . . . doesn't. I'm struggling to make sense of it, of whether there's even anything there. I think I'm coming to terms with a new sense of spirituality. I don't have to hold so tightly to the Bible. Religion doesn't have to consume me. Maybe that's heresy, but it's where I'm at.

DURING

I am his chosen prophet. He talks to me and me alone. Nothing else matters.

I am nine years old when a teacher asks whether I'd like to keep other kids safe. I will be called a safety patroller, helping direct traffic in the minutes before school began. Of course, it's a ceremonial position, and the adults do most of the actual work. But my new job means everything to me. I wear a bright green belt that signals to my peers and the grown-ups around me that I am not just any kid but a role model. I wish I could wear the belt everywhere.

I hope other students look at me with envy, but that isn't all. At heart, I feel lucky to be wanted, to be chosen. To be special. Isn't that what most of us are chasing, anyway? When your boss shouts you out or a stranger compliments your outfit and you get a tingle in your stomach that assures you, yes, you have done something right, even if it's as small as picking the blue shirt instead of the red one or turning in a spreadsheet with time to spare, it's one of the loveliest parts of the human experience.

Sure, it's nice to be on safety patrol or to get invited to an ice-cream social for surpassing a reading goal, but it leaves me lacking. I need to be extraordinary in a different way. All I want is for God to start talking. I know he can do it because the Bible tells me, and everyone at church hears all sorts of stuff. Whenever I lie, I cross my fingers that God won't reveal my misstep to my pastor. He does that, you know. Sometimes, God tells your dirty secrets to a person praying for you, and they'll whisper what he said so only you can hear. Or he'll send a dream and expose your sins to someone that way. Even your thoughts can send you to hell if they're bad enough.

I don't want to hear from him for gossip's sake, although it would thrill me if he shared details about everyone else's transgressions. I need him to talk about why the panic attacks that have plagued me for years aren't getting better. The platitudes that once satisfied me no longer work. He works in mysterious ways—so what? Is that a reason for him to ignore me? For a God who the Bible tells me is kind and compassionate, he doesn't seem to care very much. I need him to speak to me if I'm going to keep believing in him. I present this threat in my prayers with conviction. Surely, if he cares, he will answer.

No dice.

On the good days, I allow myself to think he is responding subtly, through someone checking on me when I'm having a hard time or with a beautiful rainbow after a storm. When life is grim, I am angry. Perhaps I'm missing the signals or not praying hard enough. Should I speak in tongues more furiously? Is fifteen minutes with my eyes tightly closed, muttering quietly, enough? Would more time convince him to take me seriously?

Does it matter?

I run through the halls of the unit, feeling like I may explode from the energy coursing through my veins. There's a song I regarded with indifference when it became popular last year, but now it's the only thing on my mind. "WAYMAKER MIRACLE WORKER PROMISE KEEPER," I scream. My knees give out as I sing. The other patients look at me. A nurse asks whether I want to lie down for a few minutes.

GOOD. This is what God wants. The world will see me and know that he is real.

How did I ever hesitate? I would give anything for access to the old Bible for inspiration, but the new one I'm writing will have to do. I try to recall the Scriptures I memorized as a child, but I'm coming up short. Only one comes to mind. I scrawl out the words of Acts 2:38 in my notebook: "Repent and be baptized, every one of you, in the name of Jesus Christ for the forgiveness of your sins. And you will receive the gift of the Holy Spirit." I'm unsure what it means, but God wants it in the New Bible, so it's staying. He's the one in charge, after all.

When I think about how much he loves me, I have no choice but to weep. It's unlike anything I've known before. I am devastated for anyone who's never experienced this. Of course, I'm Jesus, so no one will ever feel his blessings as profoundly as I do—but everyone has access to some extent. I don't know much, but I'll never leave this behind.

He's just too good.

TWO DAYS AFTER

It is my second night home from the hospital. I am so tired, but my body feels like it's covered in ants if I stay still. I am not prepared for how hard it is to rest. The urge to move is killing me. Finally, I pull my gray weighted blanket from the closet and force myself to get in bed. It pains me to take a break from pacing, but my feet are tired from all the movement. I wish I had a fitness tracker to count my steps. I would've hit ten thousand without a problem with all my walking. I curl into a ball without any distractions—for once, I am not staring at my phone.

My husband handed it to me when I asked for it earlier, but I gave it back after a few minutes. The bright light is too harsh, and my social media feeds are too overwhelming. I'm not ready yet. With time, I'll assume my usual routine of obsessively switching between Facebook, Instagram, Twitter, and Reddit. My weekly screen time report will eventually embarrass me again. But not today.

I inhale deeply, willing myself to actually drift off to sleep, but I'm creeped out by how quiet it is in the room. I wonder whether white noise would provide some relief. I consider asking my husband to return my phone so I can find a calming video. For some reason, I don't feel it'll help. Things are so silent that I'm tempted to start pacing again. Or maybe I'll play music? I can't place why I feel this way. But then, it hits me.

I miss God.

My problem isn't fixable with an app that blares static sounds or meditative prompts. The reason the silence bothers me is deeper than that. It's the first time in weeks that I'm not dozing off with God whispering in my ear. Over the past few days, I've had to stop myself from asking him for advice. Old habits die hard, I guess. It feels unhinged to think, but . . . I wish he was still here.

I hate to even say it. He showed me terrible things I'll never forget—people dying, children being abused, my loved ones attacking my daughter. For his sake, I humiliated myself. But, I remind myself, none of it was God. It was all my mind playing tricks on me. I don't know why I'm longing for the revelations—almost craving psychosis again. I do my best to ignore the idea. What does it say about me that I'm chasing a high only trauma can bring?

The episode destroyed me—I know this to be true. So why can't I get over the nagging feeling that something is missing? I'm wide awake now, no longer trying to fall asleep. Before everything went south, I hadn't prayed in a long time. So what do I do now? I open my mouth and try to form a prayer. The words feel foreign on my tongue. Abruptly, I stop. God has told me enough. I don't need anything else from him.

THIRTEEN YEARS BEFORE

It's my freshman year of high school, and I am obsessed with a boy who plays on our school's soccer team. Guys don't pay attention to me, so I do my best to brush it off and ignore how my stomach flutters when we talk between classes. Then, I hear it through the grapevine (*Tyler said that Julie said that Jessica said . . .*) that he might like me, too. Thrilled doesn't even begin to cover it. I was going to be a girlfriend.

I take my new role very seriously. My Myspace profile picture quickly changes, and I give him the coveted first spot in my top eight friends. I can add music to my profile, and I choose "Bubbly" by Colbie Caillat. Is this what it feels like to be in love?

Alas, our romance quickly fizzles for the usual reasons fourteen-year-old children don't make it to the altar. I am devastated, but I do my best to take it in stride. When I spot him in the hallway, I turn around. Our friends congregate by our lockers between classes, but I artfully dodge everyone. Eventually, summer comes, and our short-lived fling is forgotten by all. My next relationship ends in marriage; our biggest fight lasts one day. I still know a thing or two about breakups, though. I've grieved nonromantic relationships, and the pain is the worst.

Justified, unfair, expected, out of the blue—I've lived it all. Sometimes, we drift apart naturally as the text messages become less playful and more formal. Someone I thought I'd grown close to once let me know she viewed our relationship much differently from how I did. Regrettably, I bawled. At least once, I discovered a friendship was over after realizing they'd unfollowed me on Instagram.

The intensity with which I mourn these lost relationships borders on histrionics. Wondering where I went wrong, I shed enough tears to leave my eyes red and puffy. On my worst days, I wonder why anyone would ever want to be friends with me in the first place. To stop talking to someone you've known intimately is a unique, complicated pain that's nearly impossible to explain to someone who hasn't lived it.

And then there's my conundrum. Nothing I've experienced compares to what I'm currently going through. What if the other person isn't a person at all? If you're mourning someone who isn't even *someone*? When I think about how much I miss the voice, the longing is so intense it feels like it'll kill me. I try to beat the truth into myself. *It wasn't even real! It ruined your life!* But the allure is too fierce to fully let go. Much like a dream that leaves you disoriented because you would've sworn that it was happening in real life, the sudden end to my infatuation with God hits me hard. One day, he reveals the world's secrets to me so quickly that I can barely keep up. On the ward, my fellow patients love my prophecies; at least, that's what my mind tells me. Days later, my thoughts are uncomfortably silent. My experience was authentic to me, but not real for anyone else.

I allow my mind to roam to the idea I'm afraid to speak aloud. The seed has been planted, and I can no longer ignore the thought. A tiny part of me—at least I hope it is small—wonders whether the medications are hindering me from something I should have. I furiously try to brush it off. Remember, I tell myself, you don't actually want this. There's no need for your mind to tell you anything. It wasn't divine intervention. You just want to feel special.

If I say it enough, I'll start to believe it.

TEN YEARS BEFORE

When I am seventeen, I look at my college acceptance letters and feel overwhelmed. Multiple schools have expressed interest, and I cannot decide which would be best for me. So I pray. Weeks go by and I repeat the same desperate prayer. *God, this is going to change my life. I need you to show me the right way.* He never talks back. In the end, common sense wins, and I pick the university with the biggest financial aid package. I wonder which would be worse: If God can respond but leaves me alone when I need him most or if he isn't there. The possibilities terrify me, and I bury the thought.

Here's the problem. God is endlessly loving and wants the best for me, but he only talks when he feels like it, which is never. You can trot out explanations for why this is—I try plenty myself—but none of them feel particularly satisfying. Maybe it makes me a bad person to wonder, but I can't help but think about it. He doesn't owe me anything, but I have promised him a life full of devotion, and then for eternity once I die. Something in return would be nice.

Two years after the "where should I go to college" prayers, I visit a church a few miles from campus. As the music swells, I feel a push to share something with the girl beside me. I awkwardly turn and tell her that God has something he wants her to know. She nods, receptive to my wild introduction. I put my hand on her shoulder, and the words spew out. She's been struggling and looking for signs that everything will work out. I whisper loudly to be heard over the song pulsing through the building. God has a plan for her life and wants her to know she's loved. I pull away, and she thanks me. I realize there are tears in her eyes and feel proud of myself for listening to his voice. For once, he is saying things, and I am helping people.

Years later, when I am a much more cynical version of myself, I view the interaction in a new light. My impossibly vague prophetic word could've applied to everyone in the room. Aren't we all having a hard time in one way or another? Why give God credit for something my mind came up with on its own? I wonder whether I gained more from the interaction than the girl did. Sure, she seemed emotional, but we were in an environment designed to elicit the tears she shed—soft piano and dimmed lights, everyone speaking in gentle tones. Who knows whether any of it was real or manufactured? Looking back, I am embarrassed by the whole night, me hearing from God and deciding to tell her. Maybe he does talk to people, but I am not one of them.

Until psychosis.

TEN MONTHS AFTER

I flop on the futon in my office, open the Instagram app, and idly scroll through unread messages. I have a work project due tomorrow that I am valiantly procrastinating on starting. I work best under pressure, I think. No point in beginning today. Future Ayana will almost certainly hate me for this, but whatever. A message pops up from an unfamiliar name, and I curiously tap it.

"Hi, Ayana, this is random, but are you writing a book or considering it?"

I roll my eyes. Is there a multilevel marketing scheme to recruit aspiring writers now? I have no dreams of becoming an author, and I tell her as much. She responds nearly immediately, and my stomach tightens as I read the message.

"This may be weird or random, but I have a gift from God where I see visions. Yesterday, I saw you as a best-selling author of a book, I'm not sure what about . . ." The DM ends with her thanking me for my work and asking God to bless me for all I do. To put it plainly, I'm creeped out. Her words mirror what I heard at the start of my psychotic episode. That's weird, right?

That's the tricky thing about prophetic words purportedly from heaven. They're most believable when they're vague. When someone says you'll overcome your current struggles because God has a unique plan for your life, it's generalized enough to apply to 99 percent of the population. Getting more specific—say, declaring someone's future profession or detailing particular ways their life will change—is risky. When I was heavily involved in the church, I heard it all.

I think back to a few years ago when I stumbled upon an article about a televangelist who drew in thousands with hyperspecific prophecies, reciting people's names and addresses thanks to his gift from God. Eventually, the truth came out—he wore an earpiece, and his wife fed him information from backstage. Before the exposé, he was pulling in millions in donations. Charlatans abound.

Talking to God and making money off it is an easy scam, but I don't think everyone who says they've received a revelation is trying to con you. Aren't we all looking for connection and finding it in different ways? If you've longed to make a difference your entire life, prophesying isn't a bad way to do it. Not only do you get to communicate with the divine, but you can also comfort people with the words you receive, like the woman who messaged me.

I tap her profile, wondering what I'll find, but leave disappointed. She offers no indicators of a special connection to heaven on her Instagram account. It's a coincidence, a perfect example of a broken clock being right twice daily. I remind myself that this woman could've messaged dozens of people the same thing. Maybe she did. But this is unnerving for a reason I can't quite place. At least I know she got it wrong.

I never want to write a book.

CHAPTER TWELVE

The Evidence

Whenever she gets an idea, she jumps up, runs down the hall, and continues to write in her book.
—My Clinical Documentation Record, page 315

THE LAST DAY

Finally, it is time to leave hell—this time, I'm speaking metaphorically. I am smiling so big that my mouth hurts. They give me a paper bag to collect my belongings. Someone asks whether I want to take my handwritten books with me. I hesitate. It takes me a second to gather my thoughts. I couldn't keep up with my brilliant mind a few days ago, so I frantically wrote everything down. No revelation was too small. If you woke up the smartest person alive, wouldn't you want to write it all down, too? The stack of books is impressive. I had a lot to say. But now, the medications have slowed me, and I can't find an answer. Wouldn't it make sense to toss them? I'm not rewriting the Bible like I've told everyone on the ward—it is embarrassing to think of my life a week prior, when I insisted I was a prophet. If the journals go in the trash, I never have to think about them, and—in some ways, this experience—again. It is tempting. But I still feel attached to the books, where I recorded almost every thought for nearly three weeks. Sure, they capture a part of my life that I'd rather forget, but a lot of effort went into them. Weirdly, I feel protective of the journals. It is far from my best writing work, but I can't let it go.

I say yes.

Hours earlier, I am sitting in my room on the ward when I hear a *knock, knock, knock*. The doctor tells me the medical team thinks I've gotten all I can out of the hospitalization, and further treatment isn't needed. Instead, I'll have telehealth visits with my outpatient psychiatrist and therapist. I listen intently, trying not to get my hopes up. Standing in one place is hard for me, but I force myself to focus. Something tells me it's crucial to remain as calm as possible. She pauses before saying the words I've been cautiously expecting. "It'll take a couple of hours, but we're filling out discharge paperwork," she tells me. "We've called your family, and they'll be here when it's time." I can barely believe it. I am going home.

Visitors aren't allowed inside the building because of pandemic restrictions, so I walk out with a stranger. The man escorting me out of the hospital doesn't talk. I stay silent, too, afraid of what I may say if I open my mouth. I can't trust the unfiltered version of myself anymore. The heavy automatic door opens, and I feel the sun on my skin for the first time in almost three weeks. I usually hate sweating, but the oppressive September heat doesn't bother me today.

When we enter the parking lot, the man asks whether I see any familiar vehicles. I crane my neck but don't see any cars I recognize. My heart sinks. Who could blame my family for cutting me off after I called them cheaters and murderers? The doctor must have lied. No one is here for me. The man asks if I need an Uber or a taxi. My chest feels heavy as I start to say yes. But then out of the corner of my eye I see someone waving. It's my husband, and my father is standing next to him. My heart lifts.

I climb into the car without looking back at the hospital, where I hope to never return. As I swing my body into the seat, I nearly stop breathing. She is here, too. I'd stressed over which car seat would be best, reading countless reviews and safety ratings before settling on the one holding my daughter. I was so ready to be the parent who paid attention to every detail. Now, she stares at me unblinking for the first time in seventeen days.

My father slowly reverses the car, and my husband contorts his body to look at me from the front seat. It's hard for me to read his expression—happy but something else, too. It hits me later that he is still hurt from losing me, even though my absence was temporary. He didn't know whether I'd come back. My father tells me I can have anything I want for lunch. Complaining about the mediocre food and bitter coffee was low on my priority list at the hospital, but I'm now delighted at the thought of a hearty meal. I opt for a decaf latte from a coffee shop down the street and Italian food for dinner. I sip the drink that tastes like the best coffee I've ever had, even though it's objectively mediocre, and look down at my perfect baby. We did it. I survived the worst time of my life.

A few days later, I ask my mother to take a picture of me and her. I'm unsteady on my feet, my pants are saggy because of the weight I lost at the hospital, and my smile doesn't quite reach my eyes—but I am home.

I do not know that the hardest parts are still ahead.

When I get home, I shove the bag underneath my bed and try not to think about it. Although I want the notebooks, I also don't ever need to see them again. But it calls to me much like any vice, and I pull the bag out one night when I cannot sleep. Being in bed is hard for me because I cannot stop moving. I later learn this is called akathisia, and it's a side effect of one of my new medications.

I open the bag slowly, like something might jump out at me. My heart is racing. I don't know why I'm so scared—after all, these books kept me company for a long time. Why should I avoid them now? Something tells me to sort through the pages and decide what to throw away. My husband is stuck in front of his computer, working a late shift in our home office, and I speed-walk there in case I need help sorting. When I show him the bag, a look of concern falls on his face. I can't let it bother me. Lately, he's always worried.

I dump everything onto the colorful rug I carefully picked out during a better time. My problems used to be so simple, I think. I fretted over which pattern to buy for weeks. Now, I'm reading fantastical things I wrote during a mental break. How do you decide what to keep when none of it means anything? At first glance, I consider throwing it all away, like I should've done at the hospital. But as I keep reading, words start to jump out at me. Calling it coherent would be generous, but it makes more sense than I thought. My husband is sitting only a few feet away, but I can't tell him that I'm finding value in my writing. He's anxious enough as it is.

I put the journals and scratch paper into two piles: one for the pages I deem worthy and one for trash. I pick apart the pages, skimming my notes before deciding whether something will remain. There's no clear method to my approach. Does it resonate with me? Or is it funny? (Some of the pages make me laugh.) If so, it gets to stay. If not, I toss it to the side and make a note to take it to the recycling bin when I'm done. When I get through the pages in the bag, I stop momentarily to allow myself to think about what I've read. It feels like I might throw up. It didn't seem like it a few minutes ago, but I think I've made a mistake.

I grab a box from the garage and stuff it with the notebooks I want to keep and the clutter that littered the bottom of the bag. I shove it on top of a wire shelf in my closet, tucking it behind the purses I never carry and scarves that are only brought out a couple times a year, thanks to Florida's mild winters. As I leave the closet, I vow not to open the box again. I don't last long.

―――

Before the world hears it all, I trickle information to the people closest to me. My friends figured something was wrong when my always-online self suddenly disappeared for weeks. First, I am coy, alluding to a hard time. Only the people closest to me know the reason for my absence. The sordid details are mine until they aren't, and I decide to spill. I share a social media post discussing the hospitalization; someone attempting to read the lines would assume I'd suffered a severe depressive episode. I'm too ashamed of the psychosis to call the experience what it is.

But one day, someone asks me an in-depth question, and something changes. I don't feel like being vague anymore. I start to talk about psychosis in conversation. And I begin to consider writing about it—the only way I truly know to process. I draft an essay and read it over fifty times before pitching it to news publications. An editor from *Cosmopolitan* expresses interest, and my secret is suddenly public knowledge. And people start to listen.

I cry through interviews, speak solemnly on podcasts, and pour my heart into articles and blog posts—this is what coping looks like. If I cannot undo the psychosis, I think, I will help other people who are suffering. The goal is admirable, but I often fall short. It all exhausts me, a truth I try my hardest to ignore. Answering the same questions repeatedly, trying to explain how my life fell apart without talking too much. Seeing my trauma packaged into soundbites and reshared on Instagram. But the struggle is worth it if I can help even one person. Or maybe not.

People ask the same questions, wondering how it all began and what it's like to experience delusions. Occasionally, they scramble for something to say and struggle to find the words. Awkward silence becomes a norm. When they catch their verbal footing, they look at me with admiration. "I couldn't have gotten through it," they say. This is meant as a compliment. Making it to the other side means I'm determined and have proven something to myself. But I find myself resenting the sentiment. What were my options?

And yet, I have a similar thought. Nightmares about my husband's untimely death leave me soaked in sweat. When I see a story about someone losing their partner, I have to keep scrolling. But I feel awe at the survivor. They're stronger than I am for getting through. If it ever happens to me, I won't be able to continue living. I'm careful to never say these things aloud for fear of my insensitivity becoming known. Still, part of me thinks I'm not strong enough to deal with something that devastating. But who is? Sure, some people are probably equipped to handle misfortune, but most of us push forward because there is no other choice. The cruelty the universe doles out does not discriminate.

I am no braver than anyone else. I make space for the woman who has a hard time after giving birth, even if her experience isn't as traumatic as mine. In the same vein, my outspokenness about pregnancy loss makes me no more valiant than someone who never shares their miscarriage at all. I persist through psychosis because I have no other way. It robs me of every comfort I know. When I get home from the hospital, I must completely rebuild myself. I don't want to, but I must. I overcome the aftermath of pregnancy loss for the same reason. We are more capable of surviving the unthinkable than we believe.

TWO MONTHS AFTER

Requesting the records takes only a few minutes. I enter my name, birth date, information about my hospital stay, and a picture of my driver's license into the hospital's web portal. I pick which specific documents I want, which is all of them. Abstract summary. Check.

Progress notes. Check. Therapy notes. Check. Emergency room report. Check, check, check. I choose to have the file emailed to me. Otherwise, I'd be checking the mail multiple times a day.

It arrives in my inbox a couple of weeks later around lunchtime as I settle in to eat takeout sushi. I jump when I get the notification. I am still picking up the pieces of my shattered life weeks after my release. I need to regain control and face my problems head-on. If anything, my decision to seek out the documents is empowering. This is what I tell myself.

The sheer size of the file stuns me. It is hundreds of pages long, many irrelevant to me—bloodwork values, medication logs, reports on how I ate. The information I've been looking for is buried in the records—the notes filed at the end of each shift that vividly describe my behavior. I shudder from embarrassment when I start to read. I didn't have confidence in my medical team because I thought they were trying to kill me. My mind has allowed me to forget a lot of this, but it comes flooding back. What a nightmare.

I close out of the file as quickly as I can. I pull out my phone and mindlessly scroll, hoping to distract myself from the disturbing questions in my brain. The doctors know best. It's silly that I didn't have confidence in them.

But I still have nagging questions. I have gained significant weight in only a few weeks from the drugs—my personal hell. Any side effect is worth keeping my mind intact, right? I can only hope. With a closet full of clothing suddenly too small, I stroll the aisles of my local Goodwill searching for cheap pants that will fit and wonder whether I really need the meds.

At home, I reopen the file because I can't help it and scroll through the hospital records page by page until my hand cramps. About two hundred pages in, I stop. "She states, 'The doctor is trying to kill me with all these pills.'" My emotions are swirling so intensely that I can hardly figure out my feelings. I don't think the doctors are trying to murder anyone anymore, but I wonder whether there's a speck of truth. I came home from the hospital with six psychiatric medications that I space taking throughout the day; my bathroom counter looks like a pharmacy. I sleep so heavily that my phone's alarm no longer serves a purpose. My hands tremble when I hold a pen. The medication is supposedly keeping me sane, but at what cost? I cringe when I remember how I treated my medical team during psychosis; after all, Dr. Garza and Dr. Ramirez were looking out for me. I can trust them. They want me to recover—that's why I'm taking so many meds. But a small, scared part of me feels a niggling doubt. They could still be wrong.

What if I never get better?

THREE MONTHS AFTER

I get up from my chair to stretch. I don't know how long I've been reading my hospital records this time—Thirty minutes? One hour?—but my body is telling me it's time to take a break. My mind also sends me signals to stop, but those are easier to ignore. When I told my therapist that I'd requested my medical history and hoped to remember all I'd forgotten, she looked at me with serious eyes. "Those records are not meant for your consumption," she told me, her tone serious. I stopped myself from rolling my eyes at the dramatic response.

Admitting when I'm wrong isn't one of my strong suits, but she is onto something. I close out of the 472-page file after skimming a page that reminds me I spoke in the third person whenever God or Satan took over my body, which was often.

I close the document aptly labeled "hospital records" and make sure it's saved to the desktop. I shut my laptop so I can think; I already know I won't be finishing any more work today.

I cannot share all the things that bother me from the file, but I am struck by my level of paranoia in the hospital. This isn't my first attempt at reading the records, but it's no easier. My vivid memories are reduced to clinical jargon, and my humanity feels lessened. Hospital Ayana is rude. She accuses other people of being sent by the devil. She announces that nurses and doctors can't be trusted; when this gets old, she shifts her attention to patients who are secretly possessed.

Psychosis brings out a version of myself that I didn't know existed. I am irritable. I do not make friends wherever I go. Does it matter? After all, no one checks into a psych ward to expand their social network. Getting out is the only thing on most people's minds, but it wasn't on mine—at least in the beginning. I had bigger things to worry about than leaving. God took away all my anxiety and doubts, making me the most courageous person alive. I was invincible.

Now, I'm more scared than ever.

Returning to the real world meant I had to pick up the pieces. Things are different now.

I close my office door on the way out. That's enough for today.

FOUR MONTHS AFTER

My husband holds our daughter in his hands, their faces illuminated by the tree in our living room. This is my favorite holiday, but I want nothing to do with it now. Honestly, I'd rather be in bed on my phone. I'm so tired. Skipping it altogether would've been fine by me. It's not like she's old enough to remember. But he convinced me otherwise, so we put on a Christmas music playlist and rifle through ornament boxes as she watches intently from her bouncer. He has a knack for gently forcing me to see the good.

Now, he talks to her in a high pitch that would be grating if it weren't coming from someone I love. She babbles happily in response. I try my best to smile, but my mind is all over the place. She never looks at me like that. When he enters the room, her arms flail around as if she'll combust if he doesn't pick her up right that second. He is the preferred parent. This would be a hard pill to swallow in the best circumstances; I've never done well with second place. But now, it wrecks me. The first month of life is formative, and I was gone for almost all of it. Of course my baby doesn't want me.

I go through the motions for the rest of the night. After my husband finally falls asleep, in bed next to him I turn down the brightness on my phone and open the Reddit app. I wait till I hear snoring before I go down the rabbit hole; he would disapprove of what I'm doing, and I'm not interested in his opinion. I search for variations of "postpartum psychosis child traumatized" and "postpartum psychosis effect on child," but the responses frustrate me. They all differ, so how am I supposed to know what's true? I close out of the app and head to Google, where I quickly scan reports on how parental absence changes children. I feel validated, even though I do not like what I find.

One study examined parent–child relationships in which the mother had postpartum depression.[1] The study is twenty years old and only includes twenty-five participants. Still, the conclusion is enough to make me panic. The children of women with higher depression scores were less happy when they were reunited after separation. The study continued, "In contrast, most fathers in families where the mothers scored high on the EPDS seemed to establish joyful relationships with their children and secure child–father attachment 15–18 months postpartum, as if the father 'compensated' for the mothers' depressive symptoms."

Critical thinking disappears as I try my hardest to avoid panic. My journalism professors taught me to view everything I saw online with skepticism. The lesson followed me into adulthood—I fact-check anytime someone shares a statistic, not caring that it's probably annoying of me to not give them the benefit of the doubt. My training goes out the window when I search for proof I've irreversibly damaged my relationship with my daughter by leaving. I continue to devour academic research, looking for studies to confirm my suspicions. I hit the jackpot.

Another study examines how mother–child separation affects children in the long term. Researchers found that children younger than two separated from their mothers for more than a week are more likely to eventually show aggression.[2] The study views these separations through the lens of attachment theory, which says caregivers should be present for children to become bonded to them. Researchers found that any break, even vacation or work trips, could negatively impact small children. As I read the study, I feel a pit in my stomach. If separations for innocuous reasons can cause problems, how would a psychiatric stay affect her?

I frantically skim the paper, ignoring a sentence that should've been a comfort. "A maternal separation is quite likely not as distressing to an infant if he/she is left in the care of another attachment figure to whom he/she is securely attached." Everyone cherished the baby while I was hospitalized and in the days after. My family members stopped by daily, taking turns holding her, changing diapers, and mixing bottles of formula. One of my closest friends came over to check on my family without anyone asking. My absence was apparent, but she was far from neglected. And what were my options? Postpartum psychosis increased the risk that I'd harm her. Any good parent would remove themselves from a situation before it became dangerous. Separation was the only option for us both, as excruciating as it is to accept.

But I don't care. I've found the ammunition I need to prove what I already knew. I screenshot the most devastating bits from the academic papers and save them in a note on my phone—a file to reference anytime I feel like a good mother. I needed evidence that I've ruined my relationship with her before it began, and I've finally found it. I plug my phone in to charge and try to push away everything I've read to fall asleep, but it's too late. Instead, I toss and turn for what feels like hours, wondering why I ever thought I'd be a competent parent in the first place. Wouldn't my husband do a fine job by himself? This is the first time I wonder whether she might be better off without me. It won't be the last.

FIVE MONTHS AFTER

It is time to rummage through the box again. I don't know what I'm looking for until I open it. I reread scraps of paper I've almost committed to memory, unsure why I can't leave it all behind. I come across a notebook with "NOT SCARED" scrawled across the front, and I can't help but chuckle. I don't remember this one. Five months ago, I was bold and brave. Other people's opinions of me didn't matter.

I sit on the closet floor as I flip through the pages, trying my best to be blasé. I don't want any of this to affect me. Everyone else has moved on, so why can't I? This is why the box bothers me so much. I have tried blocking out as much as possible, but I cannot escape what happened. It always finds me.

FOUR YEARS AFTER

I skim the article on the screen in front of me, digesting the information as quickly as possible. Lindsay Clancy, a Massachusetts woman, allegedly strangled her three children in 2023 while her husband was picking up takeout food for the family. Now, a magazine has profiled him. The article found me via Reddit, and I tried to avoid clicking before giving in to temptation. Lindsay didn't have a postpartum psychosis diagnosis at the time of the murders, but her attorneys have suggested that it could've been a factor.

Once I start looking, I cannot stop. I type "Andrea Yates" into my internet browser, barely giving it time to load before I click the first result. I know what I'll find—in my early twenties, I was fascinated by true crime—but that does not make it any easier to read. In 2001, the Texas mother drowned her five children in a bathtub. I flinch as I read about the order in which she killed them. I close out of the tab and open another. I am drawn to web forums where people debate who's to blame: her husband for pressuring her to have more children, her psychiatrist for changing her medication regimen, or a friend of the family whose writings could've influenced her. Of course, the person people blame the most is Andrea herself. What kind of person kills her kids?

These stories unsettle me, but I cannot look away. And I don't want to. We are inextricably linked, and I feel a particular kinship that's only possible when you've heard the same voices. Dismissing these women as monsters is easy, and it feels natural to gasp at disturbing tabloid headlines. I understand the instinct. But it's a disservice to everyone if we ignore the truth: A person experiencing postpartum psychosis who harms their child isn't evil.

If you've never lived through it, it's impossible to fully understand how real the delusions feel. We all rely on our minds and trust our guts, and that inclination doesn't suddenly disappear when an episode starts. As a mother, I must keep my daughter safe. I'd do anything for her. The same is true for many of the postpartum psychosis survivors vilified by the media. If I'd been home and the voice told me to send her to heaven, I almost certainly would've listened. It's hard for me to finish that thought.

CHAPTER THIRTEEN

You Won't Be Here Forever

She states that she engages in self-sabotage because she is fearful of going home.
—My Clinical Documentation Record, page 255

I am always in control until I'm not.

Only other people embarrass themselves until I do.

My mind belongs to me until it doesn't.

My brain leaves me, and when it finds me again, I must piece it together. I have no choice but to tear it all down before figuring out what's next, just like you would in a home declared uninhabitable. Who is Ayana? There are the basics, of course. I love my family. Writing is the only hobby I've stuck with. My favorite colors are dark green and lilac. In a perfect world, I'd have a strawberry matcha latte in one hand and a tray of spicy tuna rolls in the other. But what does it really mean to be me beyond the information you'd find out during a work icebreaker? Hell, what does it mean to be alive?

The psychosis ruins me. It destroys all I know to be true. But I am given a unique opportunity—much like a kid running around Build-A-Bear drunk on power, I have plenty of choices as I reckon with myself. Am I a welcoming person? Before the episode, my answer would've been a confident yes. I'm not so sure anymore. I spent years yelling at anyone who would listen about the importance of eradicating the stigma surrounding mental health conditions, but there was an asterisk. If you acted embarrassingly—really, in any way society deemed unacceptable—my attitude was equal parts pity and relief that I wasn't in your shoes. Then, I became one of the people I used to ignore.

The shame of the psychosis—the delusions, the text messages, the chaos of it all—crashed with the guilt of how I would've reacted if I saw my psychotic self in public. Clutched my purse a little tighter, maybe, or moved farther along the sidewalk to increase the distance between us. My response wouldn't have been as compassionate as I would've liked to think, that's for sure. I stop to ask myself why. Would I have thought I was in danger? Fear is the only answer I can find. But really, what was there to be afraid of? No part of me would have considered the humanity of the Ayana mumbling under her breath. And I definitely wouldn't have stopped to think about what makes someone act in a way that's so unpalatable.

Now, I feel it all so deeply. The way the other patients looked at me. The awkward silence when I started opening up to people about my experience. The time a nurse mockingly agreed that all my prophecies were true, and the elation I felt before realizing she was joking. How would people on the street have treated me? The cruelty we show each other is extraordinary. Think about how many videos have gone viral of people acting bizarrely who were clearly in a mental crisis. When I used to scroll TikTok every night, my feed was filled with public meltdowns captured by people more likely to pull out their phones than ask if someone needed help. And here's the worst part—I would watch the footage of a woman's meltdown on an airplane or someone screaming at no one in particular, rarely feeling the empathy I demanded while suffering myself. We can say we're kind, welcoming, and inclusive, but how do we act when those beliefs are tested?

I've spent my entire life gripped by how I'm perceived by other people. Losing control increased the obsession tenfold. For months after the hospitalization, I agonized over every choice I made. If I felt too excited, used too many exclamation points, or had a day filled with mood swings, did that mean it was happening again?

I was psychotic for weeks, but it might as well have been years. It consumed every part of me and spit me out when finished. I have lost hundreds of hours replaying my entire life trying to determine what I could've and should've done differently.

This thought exercise doesn't provide me with much solace. It is grueling, punishing work. But it is all I know. Overthinking and dissecting my decisions are second nature. Raking myself over the coals again and again feels gratifying. I have a funny relationship with shame and how it sits in my stomach. I ask my husband to describe how I behaved in detail and share the things I may have forgotten, but he declines. I'm angry he won't indulge me.

THREE YEARS AFTER

I hold the narrow strip to the harsh fluorescent bathroom light, squinting to figure out whether I'm seeing what I think I'm seeing. It's hard to tell how many lines are on the test, so I drive to Publix to buy a digital version. I force myself to look away from the screen for five minutes. When I come back, the screen flashes a positive result. I cover my mouth to stop myself from yelling.

This is good news—great news, even. After debating for years, we decided another baby was in the cards for us. There were the usual concerns. Do we really want to pay for childcare for more than one kid? Two college funds? Isn't it wonderful that we get to sleep through the night now?

And then there are the worries that are uniquely mine. Am I willing to risk my mental health? I went to hell and back, but I got to recover on my own. Other people took care of the baby while I focused on my recovery. But now, I have an inquisitive toddler who clings to me. She'd sense if something was wrong with Mama. She's upset when I leave the room for more than a few minutes. I picture her full of questions with tears in her eyes, begging for me to come home from the hospital, and I feel dizzy. I cannot do it again. I refuse to hurt her.

Dr. Jones helps me map out all the possible outcomes, but I innately shy away from the good ones. With her help, I force myself to envision a different scenario—one that's redemptive instead of repetitive. What if this pregnancy changes me for the better?

Call it foolish optimism, but my heart wins out. Another baby is on the radar. I start taking a prenatal vitamin and pick a high-risk obstetrician who specializes in postpartum mood disorders. Dr. Garza lowers my medication dosages in case I get pregnant. Dr. Jones tells me to reach out if I get a positive test and need support. I've done everything right. I should be ready.

The excitement is there, especially when I see the smile on my husband's face, but I can't stop shaking after the novelty wears off. Isn't that how it goes? You can take every step to prepare for the big, scary thing—do all the research and read all the anecdotal responses you can find online—but it still catches you off guard when it arrives. And you wonder whether you should've gone out on a limb and left your comfort zone in the first place.

I distract myself with all the items on my mental to-do list. I text Dr. Garza, email Dr. Jones, and call my doctor's office to schedule an ultrasound in four weeks. I send my projected due date to the doula I chose well in advance. I drive to my parents' house to tell my family; I'm not great at keeping my own secrets. They scream in excitement. I try to ignore my complicated emotions, but I'm scared by the time the sun sets. The only thing on my mind is the recurrence rate of postpartum psychosis. One in two who experience the condition will have it again in subsequent pregnancies. Some say the chance is as high as 80 percent.[1] Why would anyone risk it?

Two weeks after I find out I'm pregnant, I wipe after peeing and see bright red blood. I am shaky. A frantic Google search tells me this doesn't always mean something is wrong, but I am convinced I'm losing another baby. I take our daughter to my mother and head to the hospital with my husband. After hours in the waiting room's cold chairs, they bring me back for an ultrasound. The result is inconclusive. I could be having a miscarriage, or my pregnancy could be viable. Only time will tell. I don't really pray anymore, but I decide to make an exception. The baby has to be okay. At an appointment the following week, I hold my breath until I hear the steady thrum of the heartbeat. I'm not miscarrying—at least, not right now.

Mercifully, the pregnancy continues. It hasn't hit me until now how desperately I want this baby.

―

My head feels like it weighs one hundred pounds. Staying awake is a herculean task. This is a side effect of the medication, the nurses tell me. Okay, I choke out. It feels like my mouth is full of cotton balls.

When it's my turn to talk to the psychiatrist, I tell him the medicine is working, and I don't think I'm in hell anymore. I just want to get better, I say. He seems pleased, and I know I've said the right thing. Later that day, my husband calls me. His voice sounds lighter. He says I may come home soon. We end the call with the sign-off we've used since college.

"I love you," he says.

"I love you more," I respond.

"I love you most," he finishes.

It is the first time I've told him I love him in three weeks.

After he hangs up, I go to my room to lie in the dark. A nurse stops by to ask whether I'm attending group therapy. "No, thank you," I tell her sweetly. Maybe tomorrow. I am hyperaware of my tone lately. My volatile behavior doesn't entirely embarrass me—at least, not yet—but I know it isn't getting me out of here. You catch more flies with honey, as they say. Do I remember the expression correctly? I'll have to check when I get home.

Home. A month ago, I planned to get out of the house only if absolutely necessary. I didn't want to spend any time away from my baby because I'd miss her too much. Wouldn't anybody? Besides, leaving would expose her to countless germs during the pandemic. Now, it's been such a long time—days? Weeks? I make a note to find a calendar—that I wonder whether she even knows she has a mother. And I've been surrounded by unmasked patients and workers with coronavirus running rampant. So much for me doing everything I can to protect her. I push the worries aside. At least I'm thinking clearly. COVID, the baby, wanting to google a phrase to make sure I'm not misremembering. She's real. I know she's real.

I'm almost myself again.

FOUR YEARS AFTER

I lie on a bed in a hospital gown that leaves little to the imagination. My surgery will begin any minute, and I blink away tears when a nurse tells me it's almost time. I doubt she's surprised—I can imagine most people who undergo life-altering surgery have the jitters beforehand. But the physical pain barely worries me. Am I torpedoing my life? Right now, I am in control of my mind. My daughter has a stable mother. My work is enjoyable, and our marriage is healthy. I already love my unborn son, but his birth could ruin everything.

I've spent the past eight months taking every precaution possible. Consulting with my doctor to make sure I'll get good care in the hospital. Saving to hire an overnight doula who will occasionally watch the baby overnight. Meeting with Dr. Garza to discuss what we'll do if I start to show psychotic symptoms. Limiting my access to social media so I don't humiliate myself if things go poorly. The preparation feels satisfying at the time. But now, I am hurtling toward a point of no return with no way of knowing what the outcome will look like.

The same nurse announces that they're ready for me. I say goodbye to my husband, who will join me right before the procedure begins. I quietly sob through the spinal block, the reality of the situation finally hitting me. Someone holds my hand. Someone else hangs a blue drape over my midsection. My husband is finally allowed in the operating room, holding a vomit bag up in case I get nauseous and reminding me to take deep breaths. I feel a hard tug and hear a wail. Our baby. I cradle him in my arms and cry, just like I did four years prior. He and his sister have identical birth weights down to the ounce. They wheel me to a recovery room. I feel safe here. The hospital psychiatrist checks on me twice daily. A doctor hangs a note on my door asking staff to enter only if necessary; she is concerned about how overstimulation could affect my mental health. If I go psychotic here, someone will catch it. Soon, it is time to go home, and I am on my own.

Knowing him is a joy. I watch every nap, doing my best to memorize all his features. But my anxiety is ever present. It hits me that I may think he's divine if I look at him too long, so I distract myself. I delete the Instagram app from my phone in case I'm tempted to go off on a rant. Any moment I feel too excited about my baby, I pop a benzodiazepine to calm myself down. This is one particular cruelty for me and people with similar experiences.

When you feel a rush of happiness or crushing sadness, you panic. Could it be happening again? Others can easily have a range of emotions—being down in the dumps one day and feeling incredible the next. Not us.

Happiness about a new baby is ostensibly normal, but I can't help but think of those early days with my daughter when I texted nearly everyone in my contacts and didn't feel any pain days after my C-section. When does exhilaration become dangerous? I explore the question but can't find an answer that satisfies me.

I don't exhale till the six-week mark. Most cases of postpartum psychosis start by then. I count down to the date more intently than I did for my wedding. When I look at the calendar and realize how far I've come, the worry that's clouded my judgment for over a month fizzes out. I celebrate the milestone with a latte, just like I did when I left the psychiatric hospital over four years before. For once, peace overwhelms me. The months spent planning for every outcome were worth it. I can have a baby without breaking down. My children will have a fully present parent.

I am grateful.

―

My daughter clings to me as my son plays idly by my feet. One of her favorite television shows blares in the background, and I do my best to ignore the annoying theme song. She watches in silence, her brows furrowed. I hug my baby, and he squirms out of my arms. My husband is a few feet away, cooking dinner for all of us—I have a few strengths, but none involve the kitchen.

The smell of garlic wafts in the air, and my mind wanders. Could I have pictured this future when I was lying in bed, bleeding after the miscarriage? In psychosis, when I could barely form a sentence? I feel a pit in my stomach every August, unable to place the reason till I look at a calendar and realize it's nearly the anniversary of my admission date. My body remembers what my mind blocks. But things are different now. Today, I ate breakfast, took my children to school, picked up coffee on my way home, and rushed through work to make sure I'd have enough time with the kids before bedtime. I was once afraid to dream of a life as beautifully dull as this. Parenting can be excruciating, as anyone who has raised small children will tell you. I'm quick to text my experienced friends with questions. *Do your kids ever refuse to eat? Making it through the day without an obnoxious amount of screen time—HOW? Feeling overstimulated. What should I do?* But the parts of motherhood that I'm quick to moan about suddenly feel less annoying when I remember how our journey began.

She interrupts my thoughts without looking away from the television. "Mommy," she says unprompted, "I love you." Lately, she's sounded like a big kid when she talks—not the baby I'm used to. I tickle her, and she erupts in giggles. "I love you, too," I say softly.

I remember the end of my hospital stay and a distinct moment when I felt hope. I reached for my worn notebook and a marker to write down my latest revelation. This time, it was a rallying cry that came from deep within me: "YOU WON'T BE HERE FOREVER." At the time, it was a reminder to myself that I'd eventually make it out of the hospital—or maybe out of hell. But it became so much more.

I'm no self-help guru, nor do I subscribe to toxic positivity. Sometimes, we are stuck in the mud forever. My grandmother died suddenly when I was thirty, and I felt like my grief might suffocate me. When my daughter asks innocent questions about her Grammy, I will myself not to weep. And the pain of the miscarriage sticks with me years later. I will live with the heartbreak of loss for the rest of my life, and I'm okay with the permanency of my sorrow. I honor it. How lucky am I to have known such love, even for a brief time? And, of course, the psychotic episode marked me deeply. I won't ever fully shake the residual trauma. But for me, the declaration about leaving was a well-timed reminder. The voice wouldn't always haunt me. I wasn't going to be there forever—in the hospital, in psychosis, in hell. Things were going to change, one way or another.

Even though I'm committed to kindness, I slip up—punishing myself is all too tempting. I think of the days I became furious with myself for eating a banana instead of fasting because I was desperate to reach a goal weight. Of praying for hours, convinced I wouldn't get better because of my ugly sin. Of combing through hospital records repeatedly, desperate for a reason to blame myself. The way I treat myself is sad and, frankly, unsustainable. I've reached a challenging crossroads. I can spend the rest of my days regretting every choice I've ever made. After all, even the best decisions could've technically been better. When I look at my past—childhood, psychosis, the aftermath—disappointment is easy. So many things have gone wrong, many of them out of my control. And when I became the lowest of the low, someone who folks wouldn't glance at twice, it changed me.

Something has to give. I can ruminate only so much. Some days, when all the terrible memories are looping in my head, I wonder what it would look like to come to terms with it all. Making peace sometimes feels like too optimistic a goal. But finding a way to be present? To be here instead of there. I don't know if I'll pull through any other way.

And isn't that all I can ask for? The desire to exist in the now rather than agonizing over the past or losing sleep about what's ahead? I can anguish over what I said years ago and convince myself that the worst is still to come, that it's only a matter of time before the next catastrophe. But if I take a step back and force a deep breath, the futility of all that becomes clear. That isn't a way to live. Do I *want* to get better? Chronic anxiety is a comfort. It's safer than psychosis. But why do I have to pick between those two? Is there a world where I'm allowed to just . . . be?

Maybe this is true for all of us who are too hard on ourselves. I'll never move on from the psychosis. I don't want to—it's taught me too much. But there's room in the aftermath for joy. For compassion. For life. After all, we have the privilege of being human, of living, of being changeable, of being whole.

I am whole.

ACKNOWLEDGMENTS

Missing Me wouldn't exist without the help and support of the following people, and I'm so glad for an opportunity to express my gratefulness.

Thank you to my editor, Beth Adams, for seeing the potential in this book and helping me shape it into what it became. Your thoughtful approach to my work—giving necessary feedback without ever making me feel inadequate or insecure—has helped me immensely. You have made me a better writer.

Thank you to my agent, Rachelle Gardner, for your support throughout the book-publishing process. Having someone as experienced and talented as you in my corner makes it easier for me to do this rewarding, exhausting work.

Thank you to Ashley Hong for insisting I had a book in me, even when I wasn't sure it was true. You are relentlessly encouraging and creative, cheering me on in a way that I don't feel I deserve. I wish everyone could have someone who believed in them the way you do in me.

Thank you to everyone at Worthy who helped bring this book to life. You made every step easier, and I am thankful to have a publisher with so much confidence in my work.

I am so grateful for the psychiatrists, psychologists, therapists, nurses, social workers, and other professionals who played a role in bringing me back to myself. I don't know that any of them will read this book, but if they do, I am forever indebted.

To my family, thank you for continually advocating for me when I've needed help. My life, even the hardest parts, is more bearable because of how you have protected me. Mom and Dad, thank you for catering meals for the psych ward staff when I was in psychosis. You taking care of the people who took care of me means so much.

Olivia Muenter, Haley Neer, and Gabrielle Massari—you have given me a safe space to become undone when I need to fall apart. You are the first people I tell when anything noteworthy happens, and I'm so lucky to have people who celebrate me the way you do. (And thank you for always forgiving me when I fall miserably behind on our Marco Polo chats.)

Thank you to Scott Pollenz, Michael Majchrowicz, Ashley Dye, Sara DiNatale, and Lyndsey McKenna for helping me process the most complicated things, always knowing exactly what to say during my most tired moments. Who could've known that walking into that newsroom fresh out of school would bring me you all? I'm grateful beyond measure for each of you and for our group chat—always my favorite place to drop a hot take.

Thank you to Coryn Enfinger and Megan Philp for responding to my text messages in seconds when I'm in need and always sensing if I need validation or advice. You are two of the best people I know, and it's an honor to call you my close friends. I don't know how I'd raise my kids without your guidance, love, and affirmation. I'm so glad that Watermark gave me you two.

When I met Allysar Eales on a summer day over a decade ago, I knew I'd found a forever friend, and I was right. I owe so much to you for the way you've cared for me over the years. Thank you for how you showed up for me during psychosis. When I have friends in crisis, I think about the way you loved me. You have given an example to follow.

Thank you to Tomi Obebe, Amanda Johnson, and Nicole Green for your unwavering support over the years. I trust you to bring me hilarious voice memos and the latest pop culture tweets, but it's deeper than that. Our conversations always leave me feeling less alone, regardless of the topic. And I won't ever forget the support you offered me when I was at my lowest. I love you guys.

I feel incredibly fortunate that my work has allowed me to connect with people all over the world, many of whom have told me they kept me in their thoughts and prayers while I was suffering. Thank you for every message, comment, and encouraging word. I carry them with me.

To my children, I could write an entirely different book on how loving you has transformed me. I hope I have made you proud.

And to my husband, Vagner Lage. You have carried me through so much with such grace and quiet strength. This book wouldn't have happened without your gentle encouragement, your willingness to hold me tight while I wept, and your ability to make me smile during painful moments. I wouldn't have survived without your determination to see me well again. I love you, I love you, I love you most.

NOTES

Chapter One My Broken Brain
1. "Panic Disorder," National Institute of Mental Health, https://www.nimh.nih.gov/health/statistics/panic-disorder.

Chapter Two Miracles
1. Ohio State University, "Feeling Angry? Say a Prayer and the Wrath Fades Away, Study Suggests," ScienceDaily, March 22, 2011, https://www.sciencedaily.com/releases/2011/03/110321134714.htm.
2. Matthew Thorpe and Rachael Ajmera, "12 Science-Based Benefits of Meditation," Healthline, August 15, 2024, https://www.healthline.com/nutrition/12-benefits-of-meditation.
3. Chittaranjan Andrade and Rajiv Radhakrishnan, "Prayer and Healing: A Medical and Scientific Perspective on Randomized Controlled Trials," *Indian Journal of Psychiatry* 51, no. 4 (2009): 247, https://doi.org/10.4103/0019-5545.58288.

Chapter Four The Worst Day
1. "Miscarriage," March of Dimes, last reviewed October 2024, https://www.marchofdimes.org/find-support/topics/miscarriage-loss-grief/miscarriage.
2. Jonah Bardos, Daniel Hercz, Jenna Friedenthal, Stacey A. Missmer, and Zev Williams, "A National Survey on Public Perceptions of Miscarriage," *Obstetrics & Gynecology* 125, no. 6 (2015): 1313–1320, https://doi.org/10.1097/aog.0000000000000859.
3. "Understanding Miscarriage Prevention," WebMD, November 16, 2024, https://www.webmd.com/baby/understanding-miscarriage-prevention.
4. "Miscarriage," Mayo Clinic, September 8, 2023, https://www.mayoclinic.org/diseases-conditions/pregnancy-loss-miscarriage/symptoms-causes/syc-20354298.
5. "Encephalocele," Birth Defects, Centers for Disease Control and Prevention, November 1, 2024, https://www.cdc.gov/birth-defects/about/encephalocele.html.
6. Weiyi Huang, Robin Page, Theresa Morris, S. C. Ayres, Alva O. Ferdinand, and Samiran Sinha, "Maternal Exposure to SSRIs or SNRIs and the Risk of Congenital

Abnormalities in Offspring: A Systematic Review and Meta-Analysis," *PLOS One* 18, no. 11 (2023): e0294996, https://doi.org/10.1371/journal.pone.0294996.

Chapter Five A Mother's Love

1. Katy B. Kozhimannil, Rachel R. Hardeman, Fernando Alarid-Escudero, Carrie A. Vogelsang, Cori Blauer-Peterson, and Elizabeth A. Howell, "Modeling the Cost-Effectiveness of Doula Care Associated with Reductions in Preterm Birth and Cesarean Delivery," *Birth* 43, no. 1 (2016): 20–27, https://doi.org/10.1111/birt.12218.

2. Latoya Hill, Alisha Rao, Samantha Artiga, and Usha Ranji, "Racial Disparities in Maternal and Infant Health: Current Status and Efforts to Address Them," Kaiser Family Foundation, October 25, 2024, updated November 4, 2024, https://www.kff.org/racial-equity-and-health-policy/issue-brief/racial-disparities-in-maternal-and-infant-health-current-status-and-efforts-to-address-them/.

3. Latoya Hill, Alisha Rao, Samantha Artiga, and Usha Ranji, "Racial Disparities in Maternal and Infant Health: Current Status and Efforts to Address Them," https://www.kff.org/racial-equity-and-health-policy/racial-disparities-in-maternal-and-infant-health-current-status-and-efforts-to-address-them/.

4. Janice Sabin, "How We Fail Black Patients in Pain," Association of American Medical Colleges, January 6, 2020, https://www.aamc.org/news/how-we-fail-black-patients-pain.

5. Serena Williams, "How Serena Williams Saved Her Own Life," *ELLE*, April 5, 2022, https://www.elle.com/life-love/a39586444/how-serena-williams-saved-her-own-life/.

Chapter Six I Got Lucky

1. Justyna Michalczyk, Agata Miłosz, and Ewelina Soroka, "Postpartum Psychosis: A Review of Risk Factors, Clinical Picture, Management, Prevention, and Psychosocial Determinants," *Medical Science Monitor* 29, no. 1 (2023): e942520, https://doi.org/10.12659/MSM.942520.

2. "Mother and Baby Units," Action on Postpartum Psychosis, https://www.app-network.org/get-help/mother-and-baby-unit/.

Chapter Twelve The Evidence

1. M. Edhborg, W. Lundh, L. Seimyr, and A. M. Widström, "The Parent–Child Relationship in the Context of Maternal Depressive Mood," *Archives of Women's Mental Health* 6, no. 3 (2003): 211–216, https://doi.org/10.1007/s00737-003-0020-x.

2. Kimberly Howard, Anne Martin, Lisa J. Berlin, and Jeanne Brooks-Gunn, "Early Mother–Child Separation, Parenting, and Child Well-Being in Early Head Start Families," *Attachment & Human Development* 13, no. 1 (2011): 5–26, https://doi.org/10.1080/14616734.2010.488119.

Chapter Thirteen You Won't Be Here Forever

1. Susan Hatters Friedman, Eric Reed, and Nina E. Ross, "Postpartum Psychosis," *Current Psychiatry Reports* 25, no. 2 (2023), https://doi.org/10.1007/s11920-022-01406-4.

ABOUT THE AUTHOR

Ayana Lage is a blogger and freelance writer with bylines in *The Washington Post, Cosmopolitan, Glamour,* and more. She has a BS in journalism from the University of Florida. When she's not working, you'll find her exploring her hometown of Tampa with her husband and two children.